The Challenge of Health Sector Reform

The Role of Government in Adjusting Economies

General Editor: **Professor Richard Batley, International Development Department, School of Public Policy, University of Birmingham**

Over the last two decades there has been a strong emphasis on reducing the role of government and on reforming traditional public sector bureaucracies. The new conventional view has become that, where possible, services should not be provided directly by government but be contracted out or privatized. Where this is not possible, the predominant view has been that the public sector itself should change by setting up semi-autonomous agencies and by making public management more performance- and customer-oriented.

This series investigates the application of such reforms in Africa, Asia and Latin America. Underlying the enquiry is the question whether reforms which were initially conceived in countries such as Britain and New Zealand are appropriate in other contexts. How much sense do they make where levels of public management capacity, market development, resources, political inclusiveness, legal effectiveness, political and public economic stability are quite different?

To investigate these issues, the series covers four service sectors selected to be representative of types of public sector activity – health care, urban water supply, agricultural marketing services and business development services.

Titles include:

Anne Mills, Sara Bennett and Steven Russell
THE CHALLENGE OF HEALTH SECTOR REFORM
What Must Governments Do?

The Role of Government in Adjusting Economies
Series Standing Order ISBN 0–333–94618–9
(*outside North America only*)

You can receive future titles in this series as they are published by placing a standing order. Please contact your bookseller or, in case of difficulty, write to us at the address below with your name and address, the title of the series and the ISBN quoted above.

Customer Services Department, Macmillan Distribution Ltd, Houndmills, Basingstoke, Hampshire RG21 6XS, England

The Challenge of Health Sector Reform

What Must Governments Do?

Anne Mills
Professor of Health Economics and Policy
Health Policy Unit
London School of Hygiene and Tropical Medicine

Sara Bennett
Lecturer
Health Economics and Financing Programme
Health Policy Unit
London School of Hygiene and Tropical Medicine

Steven Russell
Lecturer
Development Studies Group
University of East Anglia

with

Nimal Attanayake

Charles Hongoro

V. R. Muraleedharan

and

Paul Smithson

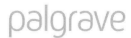

First published 2001 by
PALGRAVE
Houndmills, Basingstoke, Hampshire RG21 6XS and
175 Fifth Avenue, New York, N. Y. 10010
Companies and representatives throughout the world

PALGRAVE is the new global academic imprint of
St. Martin's Press LLC Scholarly and Reference Division and
Palgrave Publishers Ltd (formerly Macmillan Press Ltd).

ISBN 0–333–73618–4

This book is printed on paper suitable for recycling and
made from fully managed and sustained forest sources.

A catalogue record for this book is available
from the British Library.

Library of Congress Cataloging-in-Publication Data
The challenge of health sector reform : what must governments do? / Anne
Mills, Sara Bennett, Steven Russell, with Nimal Attanayake ... [et al.].
    p. cm.
  Includes bibliographical references and index.
  ISBN 0–333–73618–4
   1. Health care reform—Developing countries. 2. Medical policy–
–Developing countries. 3. Public health—Developing countries. I. Mills,
Anne. II. Bennett, Sara. III. Russell, Steven, 1966–
  RA395.D44 C435 2000
  362.1'09172'4—dc21
                                                              00–041486

10   9   8   7   6   5   4   3   2   1
10 09 08 07 06 05 04 03 02 01

Printed and bound in Great Britain by
Antony Rowe Ltd, Chippenham, Wiltshire

Contents

List of Tables

List of Figures

List of Boxes

List of Acronyms and Abbreviations

ADB   Asian Development Bank
APVVP   Andhra Pradesh Council for Hospital Management
BOI   Board of Investment (Thailand)
BOR   Bed Occupancy Rate
DFID   Department for International Development (UK) (formerly ODA)
DOSW   Department of Social Welfare (Zimbabwe)
GDP   Gross Domestic Product
GNP   Gross National Product
GMOA   Government Medical Officers Association (Sri Lanka)
GOI   Government of India
HFA   Health For All
IADB   Inter American Development Bank
IEC   Information, education, communications
IMF   International Monetary Fund
KATH   Komfo Anokye Teaching Hospital, Kumasi, Ghana
KBTH   Korle Bu Teaching Hospital, Accra, Ghana
IP   Inpatient
KHCFP   Kenya Health Care Financing Project
LIC   Low Income Card (Thailand)
MOF   Ministry of Finance
MOH   Ministry of Health
MOHCW   Ministry of Health and Child Welfare (Zimbabwe)
MOPH   Ministry of Public Health (Thailand)
NHIF   National Hospital Insurance Fund (Kenya)
NPM   New Public Management
NGO   Non-government organisation
ODA   Overseas Development Administration (now DFID)
PPP   Purchasing Power Parity
SDF   Social Development Fund (Zimbabwe)
SJGH   Sri Jayarwardenapura General Hospital (Sri Lanka)
TNBCS   Tamil Nadu State Blindness Control Society
TNMSC   Tamil Nadu Medical Supply Corporation
TNSACS   Tamil Nadu State Aids Control Society
UNDP   United Nations Development Programme
OP   Outpatient
USAID   United States Agency for International Development

Preface

This book originates from a research programme funded by the Economic and Social Committee on Research (ESCOR) of the Department for International Development (DFID). The facts presented and views expressed are those of the authors and do not necessarily reflect the views of DFID.

The research programme involved five British research groups: the International Development Department of the School of Public Policy, University of Birmingham; the Health Economics and Financing Programme, Health Policy Unit, London School of Hygiene and Tropical Medicine; the Overseas Development Group of the School of Development Studies, University of East Anglia; the Water Engineering and Development Centre of Loughborough University of Technology; and the Department of City and Regional Planning, the University of Wales. Overall coordination was provided by Richard Batley of the International Development Department, University of Birmingham.

The research on the health sector was jointly developed and planned by Sara Bennett, Anne Mills and Steven Russell. After an initial literature review of institutional and economic perspectives on government capacity to assume new roles in the health sector, country case studies were planned, with the lead being taken in Ghana by Anne Mills, in Sri Lanka and Zimbabwe by Steven Russell, in India by Sara Bennett, and in Thailand by all three. Country collaborators in the case studies were Paul Smithson and A. Asamoa-Baah in Ghana, Charles Hongoro, Philemon Kwaramba and Sifiso Chikandi in Zimbabwe, V. R. Muraleedharan in India, Nimal Attanayake in Sri Lanka, and Viroj Tangcharoensathien and Anuwat Supachutikul in Thailand. User surveys, which included views on health, were done by Carole Rakodi in Ghana and India, Tudor Silva, Steven Russell and Carole Rakodi in Sri Lanka, and Dorothy Mutizwa-Mangiza in Zimbabwe.

This book has been written by Anne Mills, Sara Bennett, and Steve Russell, with Sara Bennett taking the lead on Chapters 1, 2, 7 and 8; Anne Mills on Chapters 3, 6 and 9; and Steven Russell on Chapters 4 and 5. Nimal Attanayake, Charles Hongoro, V. R. Muraleedharan and Paul Smithson participated in a workshop to review and discuss drafts of Chapters 4–7, reviewed and commented on the entire manuscript, and provided further information to support the comparative analysis. Anne Mills edited and finalised the entire volume.

We are most grateful to all the individuals who supported the country studies, and also to Andrew Cassells, Ken Grant, Mark Pearson and Jane Pepperall who formed a steering committee for the health sector research. We also gratefully acknowledge the contribution to our thinking of our colleagues in the Health Economics and Financing Programme who are engaged in related research, notably Lucy Gilson, Lilani Kumaranayake, and Barbara McPake. The Health Economics and Financing Programme receives a work programme grant from the UK Department for International Development.

About the Authors

Anne Mills is Professor of Health Economics and Policy and Head of the Health Economics and Financing Programme at the London School of Hygiene and Tropical Medicine.

Sara Bennett is a Lecturer in the Health Economics and Financing Programme at the London School of Hygiene and Tropical Medicine, and currently based in Tbilisi, Georgia.

Steve Russell was a Research Fellow in the Health Economics and Financing Programme at the London School of Hygiene and Tropical Medicine at the time of the research, and is now completing a PhD at the LSHTM.

Nimal Attanayake is Senior Lecturer and Co-ordinator of the Health Economics Study Programme (HESP) at the Department of Economics, University of Colombo, Sri Lanka.

Charles Hongoro is a Medical Research Officer working in the Public Health Unit at the Blair Research Institute, Ministry of Health and Child Welfare, Zimbabwe.

V.R. Muraleedharan is Associate Professor of Economics at the Department of Humanities and Social Sciences, Indian Institute of Technology, Madras.

Paul Smithson is Health Sector Policy and Systems Adviser at the Department for International Development.

1
Health Sector Reform and the Role of Government

1. Introduction

There has been much substantive debate about the appropriate role of government during the past decade. While initially much of this debate took the form of a very polarised discussion of the strengths and weaknesses of government, in recent years the debate has become more nuanced. Analysts have explored the extent to which ownership alone can influence performance, and the extent to which a competitive environment or an effective regulatory framework affects the desirability of government involvement. Services have been broken down into constituent components, some more suitable than others for government provision. Current analyses of the role of government recognise that there are likely to be failures in both government and private markets. In the health sector, it is clear that while governments have made many significant achievements, including improving infant mortality rates, rapidly increasing trained local health staff and expanding health services to rural areas, there are also common negative aspects to government performance (Bennett, Russell and Mills 1996, Mills 1997a, World Bank 1987, World Bank 1993). Traditional public sector bureaucracies are often plagued by a multiplicity of problems which, in the health sector, manifest themselves in inefficient, inequitable, unresponsive and poor quality public health services.

Explanations of government failure are many and take different starting points. Many programmes aiming to improve government performance start with the most easily addressed element of capacity, that is the skills of people employed within government. Weak management skills may be particularly problematic in the health sector where the dominant role of the medical profession in decision-making can generate both inefficient and inequitable consequences (Jackson and Price 1994). Medically-trained staff often have limited management training (Mills 1997a) and limited technical skills for planning.

The behaviour of public sector employees cannot be understood without reference to the organisations and systems within which they work. Health sector bureaucracies in developing countries have been accused of being overcentralised, distancing decision-making power from communities, reducing accountability and resulting in health services which do not reflect local needs or preferences. Highly centralised budgetary and planning systems result in lack of managerial autonomy and an inability to make decisions which ensure efficient resource use. The lack of clear organisational goals and mission are also common problems (Grindle 1997, Jackson and Price 1994, World Bank 1997a) which reduce both motivation and accountability of managers.

Neo-liberal perspectives suggest that lack of competition is one of the key problems in the public sector. In the absence of the disciplinary powers of the market, slack and wasteful practices may arise and providers (unconsciously or consciously) lower the quality and quantity of services. Sheltered from competition, managers and health professionals do not face the consequences of their resource use decisions. Sheltered from the consequences of user choice, they may be more interested in improving their lifestyles and working conditions than in being accountable to users and meeting their needs.

In turn, the way in which bureaucracies operate cannot be understood (or easily changed) without reference to the broader societal relations and institutional conditions within which they are embedded. For example, lack of managerial autonomy often stems from political concerns to prevent the pursuit of controversial decisions, or to direct resources to particular projects or areas. In many developing countries the state has been criticised for being predatory and patrimonial rather than service-oriented (AM90s 1994). In the health sector it is said to have weakened civil society and stifled private and community initiatives; allocated resources according to political and bureaucratic criteria (rent-seeking) rather than efficiency or equity goals; lacked the legitimacy or instruments to pursue its plans; and disempowered local communities and users through its centralised and unaccountable relationship with the general population. Key decision-makers in the sector may identify more closely with wealthier, urban consumers, who are likely to reinforce doctors' preferences for high-technology hospital care, at the expense of meeting the needs of the poor.

Many explanations for these broader problems of governance in developing countries are rooted in the legacy of the colonial state

(AM90s 1994, Cammack 1988). At independence the state was over-extended, centralised and authoritarian in structure with few organic links with civil society and therefore limited political legitimacy or accountability (Cammack 1988). After independence the centralised state and its bureaucracies expanded: health care, education and jobs were provided by the state to help build a 'nation' (Anderson 1983) and to provide a basis of legitimacy and support for political leaders. These processes are said to have contributed to the development of neo-patrimonialism within administrations as state leaders built a web of support through patronage.

During the relatively affluent years of the 1960s and early 1970s the structural inefficiencies developing in many bureaucracies went unheeded, but international recession during the mid-1970s and 1980s resulted in a declining resource base for governments particularly in many developing countries. Simultaneously there was an ideological shift in several industrialised countries resulting in new philosophies about the appropriate role for government. Growing concerns on the part of influential external actors such as the international financial institutions and national policy-makers in developing countries about the cost and equity of health care systems, combined with an ideological shift in the West, led to a movement for reforming the role of government in health care.

2. Health sector reform and New Public Management

The current wave of interest in changing the policies, practices and management systems within the health sector is often referred to as 'health sector reform'. Health sector reform has been described as *'sustained, purposeful change to improve the efficiency, equity and effectiveness of the health sector'* (Berman 1995).

The most widespread elements of health sector reform include:

- restructuring of public sector organisations (including decentralisation and bureaucratic commercialisation whereby publicly owned facilities are restructured so that they run more along the lines of privately owned establishments: in the health sector this is usually termed hospital 'autonomy' or 'corporatisation');
- changing the way in which resources are allocated and paid to both organisations and individuals – generally with the aim of creating a clearer link between performance and reward;
- encouraging greater plurality and competition in the provision of health care services through policy measures such as liberalising the

private health sector, and contracting with or subsidising private health providers;
- seeking increased financing for health care from non-tax revenue sources such as user fees, social health insurance and private health insurance;
- increasing the role of the consumer in the health system through enhancing the power and scope of consumer choice and making health providers more accountable to community-based organisations such as hospital boards.

The diversity of reforms makes it very difficult to classify countries as 'reformers' or 'non-reformers': during the 1990s most countries, both industrialised and developing, have implemented at least some of the measures identified above. A few industrialised countries, such as the UK and New Zealand, have embarked upon ambitious programmes of reform encompassing virtually all of the measures listed (with the notable exception of financing). Similarly, many countries in Eastern Europe and the former Soviet Union have implemented far-reaching reforms, particularly financing reform and promotion of competition, as part of the transition process (Saltman and Figueras 1997). In Sub-Saharan Africa virtually every country has undertaken some reform of the system of health financing, many have embarked upon organisational reforms within the public sector, and a few, such as Zambia, have pursued more sweeping reform programmes (Gilson and Mills 1995, Leighton 1996, UNICEF 1999). Considerable change has also been seen in some Latin American countries with an inheritance of fragmented, inequitable and inefficient health system structures, which have sought to unify or restructure systems of health financing while simultaneously creating stronger incentives, often via competition, for efficiency (Londono and Frenk 1997).

Cassells (1995) has observed that 'there is no consistently-applied, universal package of measures that constitute health sector reform', though most reformers would probably state their overall goals as improving health sector efficiency, equity and sustainability. However, despite the diversity of reform packages, there is actually a strong and in part ideologically derived agenda to the current wave of health sector reform. Measures commonly adopted do not constitute an eclectic and value-neutral set of measures. In most contexts, the health sector reform agenda is inextricably tied up with a parallel strand of reform currently being extensively discussed (if not always implemented) throughout the public sector – namely, what is called 'New Public Management' (NPM) (see Table 1.1).

Table 1.1 The relationship between health sector reform and New Public Management

Building blocks of NPM	Related NPM policies	Manifestation in the health sector
Responsibility: ensure clarity of goals and purpose.	Separate policy-making from service delivery functions.	Split of policy-making and service delivery wings of MOH (e.g. Ghana, Zambia).
	Shift locus of controls to lower level managers.	Bureaucratic commercialisation: decentralisation and autonomous/ corporatised hospitals.
	Use contracts and performance agreements to promote transparency.	Contracting and performance agreements.
Accountability: increase accountability of managers to clients.	Promote client choice.	Provider payment reform: money follows patient and user fees.
	Develop consumer charters.	Development of hospital boards, district health boards and village health committees.
Performance: create stronger incentives for good performance.	Link reward to performance.	Reform of provider payment mechanisms both for individuals and facilities.
	Strengthen feedback mechanisms.	Enhance competition through separation of purchasers and providers.
	Stimulate competition.	Encourage private sector; promote internal or quasi-markets in the public sector; encourage competitive behaviour in public and private sectors.

The core of NPM has been described as government moving from 'a concern to do, towards a concern to ensure that things are done' (Kaul 1997). While the state may play a key role in development, this role is not necessarily one of direct service provision, but rather policy-making, purchasing and regulating. Analysts have written of 'reinventing government' (Osborne and Gaebler 1992) or 'the capable state' (Hilderbrand and Grindle 1994). While NPM has a clear conceptual framework, there is not yet a fully fledged body of theory (Klages and Loffler 1998). The form which NPM has taken in different countries has varied somewhat, but a key feature is a more market-oriented, private sector-type approach to the provision of public services. During the past decade Australia, Austria, Canada, France, Japan, Portugal, the UK and USA in the industrialised world have all implemented elements of such an approach with the aim of encouraging greater efficiency and quality in government (Haque 1998).

The seeds of this book grew from questioning the feasibility and desirability in developing country contexts of actually implementing NPM in the health sector. If government is to move away from the direct provision of health services to more indirect roles such as regulating private providers, or governing a managed market, or contracting for health services, then what capacities are necessary for it to take on these complex new roles effectively, and how capable do governments appear to be in performing these new functions? Given that the core ideas of NPM originated in industrialised countries, how much sense do they make in the particular institutional and bureaucratic contexts of specific developing countries? This book focuses in particular upon implementation experiences with NPM-type reforms in the health sector: while the design and espousal of reform policies may be relatively straightforward, it is during implementation that fundamental conflicts between reform policies and the institutional structures and capacities of a country are likely to become apparent. As a consequence of such a mismatch between policies and institutions, reforms may not achieve their intended goals and may have unintended, detrimental outcomes.

The following sections of this chapter describe what neo-liberal economic theory says about the appropriate role for government in health and explains the shortcomings of this theoretical framework. Alternative frameworks are then presented and discussed. The way in which the study conceptualised and assessed capacity is then described. The final sections provide a brief overview of the structure of the study and an outline for the rest of the book.

3. The poverty of neo-liberal economics

Neo-liberal economic arguments explain the need for state intervention in terms of problems of market failure. A number of problems associated with the functioning of markets in the health sector can be identified (Bennett 1991, Donaldson and Gerard 1993)[1] and much of the debate about the appropriate role for government in the health sector centres on the severity of these problems (Birdsall and James 1992). This is an empirical question, the answer to which will differ according to the type of service under consideration, amongst other factors. A wide range of services are provided within the health sector, from immunisation against

infectious diseases to environmental health controls, and to technologi-
cally advanced treatments for heart disease or cancer. These services
exhibit different degrees of informational asymmetry, externalities and
merit goods.

The variety of services offered within the health sector has led to
attempts to classify services by economic characteristic and to suggest
appropriate modes for service delivery on this basis. For example,
Musgrove (1996) classified health activities into three domains:

- public goods such as vector control and immunisation;
- low-cost private interventions, such as treatment of respiratory tract
  infections and diarrhoea;
- high-cost private interventions, such as treatments for cancer and
  injuries.

The economic characteristics (in terms of degree of externality, exclud-
ability and rivalry, degree of informational asymmetry) of services in each
of these domains differs considerably. Musgrove suggested that governments should finance services which fall into the first domain of public
goods. In the second domain, government needs to regulate insurance to
ensure efficient and equitable access to services, while in the third domain
such regulation will need to be supplemented by government financing
for the poor.

Batley (1997) refers to this approach, which links economic characteristics to mode of service delivery, as an 'organisational design' approach: it
suggests that there are universal answers to questions about the
appropriate role for government. Although Musgrove's typology provides
an elegant normative argument, there are some clear problems with this
approach, both as an analytical framework to explain the real world and as
a prescriptive guide to appropriate policy development.

First, simply identifying the presence of market failure says little about
how best that failure may be offset. For example, government subsidy of
the poor, identified as the solution for the third domain Musgrove
discusses, leaves open the question of whether this subsidy is provided
through vouchers to the poor, through publicly provided, free or low-
priced services of a quality which attract only the poor, or through
government subsidy to a national health insurance programme.

Second, the nature and extent of market failure will depend upon
factors which are highly specific to country context. These factors include
the epidemiological profile of the country, professional ethics, the
organisation and development of the business sector, and levels of

education amongst the populace. For example, in a country where there are very strong professional ethics and a highly educated population, asymmetric information between health care provider and patient will not be as problematic as elsewhere (*ceteris paribus*) and the need for regulation may be more limited.

Third, even this adapted, more context-specific interpretation of the organisational design approach may be problematic as a basis for providing prescriptive arguments for an appropriate role for government in service provision. Highly specific, contextual factors including societal values and the current organisation of the health system closely prescribe which types of reforms will be feasible and desirable. Reforms may be influenced more by historical and political processes than by technical considerations. In the terminology of North (1990), reforms are 'path-specific': where you are now influences where you can go to and where you might want to go to.

The country case studies referred to in this book explore the nature of market failures in a country-specific manner. Researchers investigated differences in epidemiological profile and hence priority health services in the country, and the consumption characteristics of these services, the nature of the private health market and issues of monopoly, barriers to entry and imperfect information. This information was used to assess how closely the actual balance of responsibilities and roles between public and private sectors corresponded to what would be prescribed by neo-liberal economic theory. However, because of the shortcomings of this approach, the study also drew upon alternative theoretical frameworks.

4.   Alternative theoretical frameworks

The literature on appropriate roles for government now reflects many different theories: two sets of theories most relevant to the health sector are reviewed here. Each of these provides conceptual frameworks which offer some insights into appropriate approaches to reforming the public sector and the health sector in particular. These theories are used in an eclectic manner throughout the book to explain findings.

4.1   Theories of bureaucracy

While advocates of 'New Public Management' often purport to revolutionise government, elements of their argument are as old as Weber. Weber's ideal bureaucratic form set out not only the elements which NPM theorists now rile against (such as an emphasis upon hierarchical control and adherence to procedures) but also some principles which NPM espouses. For example, clarity of job roles and functions was central to Weber's understanding of the ideal bureaucracy (Weber 1946). Other elements which Weber stressed are still relevant. For example, Weber argued that the responsibilities given to a job-holder must be matched by adequate authority to perform these responsibilities, wherein authority comprises:

- formal authority – that others know your responsibilities and their reporting relationships;
- personal (interpersonal) authority – that the job-holder is able to secure co-operation from others;
- resource authority – that sufficient resources (staff, skill-mix, complementary supplies) are available to perform the task;
- expertise authority – that the job-holder has sufficient skills, knowledge and experience to carry out the responsibilities.

The absence of some of these elements of authority may partly explain the problems encountered by bureaucracies in many developing countries. The definition of capacity used by the study incorporated many of these aspects. Understanding the extent to which bureaucratic failure has occurred because of capacity weaknesses within bureaucracies, as opposed to problems intrinsic to the structure of bureaucracies, appears important in terms of defining appropriate policy responses.

Much of Weberian theory of bureaucracy was founded on the importance of an impersonal approach to government: personal contacts and preferences should not be allowed to interfere with the business of government in case they endanger the impartiality of government, and mean that government serves individual interests rather than the public good. Public choice theorists have derided the notion that it is possible for individual public sector decision-makers to keep separate their motivations in public and private spheres; instead they argue that despite bureaucratic rules and regulations, civil servants are likely to pursue their own interests. The outcome of this pursuit depends critically upon incentive structures and (as suggested by principal–agent theory – see below) whether individual goals are closely aligned with organisational goals. Such a line of reasoning often leads to a conclusion that private sector activity is innately preferable to public sector action as in the private sector, ownership is the glue cementing individual motivation to high performance. However, this is not necessarily the logical conclusion of the argument: large private sector companies also have substantial problems in ensuring that workers pursue organisational goals. Creating a stronger link between performance and reward in the public sector, as suggested by NPM, is a logical conclusion of public choice theory.

4.2   New institutional economics

New institutional economics challenges neo-liberal economic theory by questioning the assumptions the latter makes about individual behaviour (particular the rationality of individual behaviour) and by reasserting the importance of institutions in explaining economic performance (Ostrom, Schroeder and Wynne 1993). In this context 'institutions' are understood to be 'the rules of the game in a society' (North 1990); they may be formal rules or informal cultural norms; either way they shape the manner in which individuals interact with each other.

One of the core assumptions of neo-liberal economic theory is that agents possess full (perfect) information. In reality, and particularly in the health sector, this is rarely the case. Patients seek care from medical professionals whom they believe are better informed than they about the nature of their illness and appropriate treatment patterns. The services of health providers are purchased by insurance organisations and other third party payers, but the purchaser generally has very incomplete information about whether the services provided were necessary or appropriate. Government finances hierarchical health systems, but there tends to be only limited flow of information between different levels of the system.

Given the complexities of health care, it is neither practical nor desirable for all agents to be perfectly informed. Instead, institutional arrangements evolve as a result of the actions of different agents. These institutions help to reduce uncertainty and ameliorate the problems associated with informational asymmetries. For example, professional organisations certify medical personnel and provide some guarantee of the quality of care which they will deliver. North's fundamental insight, particularly relevant to developing countries, was that institutions can only change incrementally and that the way in which they change is contingent upon the relative power of different actors within society. Thus transplanting new technologies (such as new forms of paying providers or contracting for services) from one society to another is unlikely to be effective unless similar institutions and institutional capabilities exist.

Institutional economics encompasses many theories and notions relevant to the discussion, the most important of which are presented here.

Transaction costs are the costs associated with making an exchange, both *ex ante* (such as seeking out a preferred supplier, drawing up a contract) and *ex post* (such as monitoring the contractor, taking sanctions if the contract is broken). Within industrial economics, transaction cost theory has been used to cast light on the 'make or buy' decision. Where the costs associated with a transaction are particularly high it may make more sense for an organisation to produce that good or service directly (through hierarchical control mechanisms) rather than through market-based exchange.

Estimates suggest that transactions costs account for a very significant proportion of GNP in industrialised countries (North 1990). In general the more complex the good or service being exchanged, the higher transaction costs are likely to be: thus the costs associated with buying a hospital inpatient episode are likely to be higher than those associated with buying a kilo of rice. Furthermore, transaction costs will be affected by the nature of institutions within a country. For example, if there is a relatively high degree of trust amongst the parties to an exchange, then transaction costs will be lower than if there is no such trust.

The informational problems in health care have also been analysed using the lens of *principal–agent theory*. Many transactions within the health sector involve a principal delegating responsibility to an agent to act on her behalf. For example, regulatory agencies can be seen as agents for government. A physician may act as an agent for a patient, and simultaneously may act as agent for an insurance organisation or health care purchaser. Economic theory suggests that problems are likely to arise in any principal–agent relationship as the agent is tempted to pursue her own goals at the expense of those of the principal. To a certain extent these problems can be ameliorated by creating appropriate incentives for agents, and by monitoring and sanctioning of agent behaviour. However, the problems may become particularly acute when there are multiple principals for any one agent, who pull that agent in different directions (Savedoff 1998). For example, hospital physicians can be seen as agents for the patient (in which context they pursue the best possible health outcomes and processes for the patient), but they may also be seen as agents for hospital management, who can have objectives (such as cost-containment) incongruent with patient objectives.

Principal–agent relationships are unavoidable in health care: they exist in an integrated, hierarchical health system (as relationships between health workers, their supervisors, and the supervisor's bosses) as well as in more fragmented, contract-based health systems. Which constellation of principal–agent relationships is most successful depends upon highly context-specific issues. While one of the core aims of NPM is to strengthen the accountability of the agent to the principal and create incentives to bring the goals of principal and agent into closer alignment, the best approach for achieving this can be determined only by reference to a particular context. For example, deciding whether a regulatory authority should be a government body or part of a professional council depends partly upon the ease with which a government body could gain access to reliable information about provider behaviour (compared to a professional body), partly on the extent to which the objectives of a professional council are likely to be aligned with those of government, and partly on the degree of trust between government and the professional body.

New institutional economics suggests that there are three prime mechanisms for ensuring accountability: *exit* (moving demand to an alternative provider), *voice* (influencing service delivery through democratic participation) and *hierarchy* (ensuring upward accountability through the system) (Paul 1992). These different strategies are more or less appropriate depending upon the type of service. For example, where there are no economies of scale and consumers can make reasonable judgements about the quality of a service provided, creating possibilities for consumer exit (or consumer choice) may help improve government service provision. Although for most primary health care services there are only limited economies of scale, consumers often have great difficulty in judging the quality of anything other than the hotel aspects of care received. Consequently, many health economists are sceptical about how significant a role consumer choice or exit can play in ensuring accountability. Where for reasons of economies of scale it may not be possible to create consumer choice, but it is important that organisations are responsive to consumer preferences, giving consumers voice within the system may be effective. During a consultation patients are in a very weak position to question health providers, but the establishment of hospital boards or health centre committees which provide a routine channel for users to express views to health authorities seems more feasible.

These two approaches emphasising downward accountability have been espoused by the NPM agenda and contrast with traditional hierarchical control mechanisms. Again, however, empirical examination of the different institutions involved in exit, voice and hierarchy is needed to ensure that the channel of accountability chosen is really an appropriate one. For example, can voice really be effective in political systems which have traditionally excluded the weak and vulnerable?

5.   Concepts of capacity

One of the principal arguments used to promote reform of the role of government both in and outside the health sector is government's inability to deliver services in a traditional manner. It has commonly been stated that government is overstretched. Ironically, capacity issues may also be one of the dominant determinants of success in implementing New Public Management or reforming the health sector. Health sector reform may reduce the role of the state in some respects, but it also pulls government into new tasks and roles which it may be poorly equipped to perform.

Prior to reform, the core government functions within the health sector would most likely be policy setting and planning, the administration of provision and the direct provision of services. Many functions such as analysis, enforcement of rules and regulations, information provision, and establishment of alternative financing systems would clearly have been seen as part of government responsibilities, but may not have taken up much of government capacity either because they were performed to a limited extent only (as with analytical functions and information provision) or because they were relatively simple functions (as with fiscal functions). Reforms have required governments both to perform functions in a far more complex environment and to extend certain functions significantly. For example, the administration of provision in a wholly public, centrally organised system may be fairly straightforward, but once systems are decentralised, and payment and/or budgetary allocation methods are reformed, this function may become much more complex to manage.

Traditionally, discussion of 'capacity building' for development has focused upon training and personnel development (Brinkerhoff 1994). However, there is increasing recognition of the limitations of such an approach and several institutional analysts have sought to broaden the conceptual framework for understanding capacity. The various approaches used to outline and understand capacity, and that adopted by the research project, are discussed in more depth in Batley (1997). The approach used here is closely allied to that presented by Hildebrand and Grindle (1994). It considers aspects of capacity internal to key implementing government agencies, notably human resources (both skills and numbers), resource availability and the appropriateness of organisational systems and structures. The framework acknowledges that more than one actor (organisation) may commonly be involved in performing any particular task, and that co-ordination between the various actors involved is a key dimension of capacity. More broadly still, the framework considers factors external to the implementing organisation(s) which may hamper or enhance capacity. These include the public sector institutional context (such as civil service rules and regulations) and the broader societal context (including the macro-economic situation, the stability of government, and the richness of civil society).

The strength of such an approach is not only that it draws attention to wider institutional factors which may act as bottlenecks preventing successful government performance, but also that it emphasises the importance of fit between different levels of the context. For example, are systems being put in place within the Ministry of Health that are congruent with broader government rules and systems? Such a broad notion of capacity may also be problematic: capacity becomes almost synonymous with development, making empirical research into the topic very unmanageable. The country case studies undertaken combined a more detailed analysis of organisational capacity (skills, systems, physical resources) with a more superficial assessment of the impact of the broader environment upon capacity.

Further refinements can be made to this conceptual framework. First, it is often useful to distinguish between the capacity of government to perform particular functions (e.g. contract for health care) and the capacity of that particular service arrangement to deliver the desired benefits. Second, as we have suggested, capacity is task-specific. Discussion of capacities (or incapacities) needs to be clearly linked to a particular function. Third, and of considerable significance, is the fact that the concepts of capacity discussed above are all static: they form one-time snap-shots of government's ability to perform a particular task. In reality, capacity is dynamic and is likely to change over time. A key question is *how* it changes over time: is government able to learn from previous experience and adapt its behaviour accordingly? This notion of adaptive capacity accords closely with North's discussion of a society's willingness to acquire knowledge, induce innovation and take risks (North 1990).

6.   Study overview

The discussion in this book is based upon four in-depth country case studies in Ghana (Smithson, Asamoa-Baah and Mills 1997), India (Bennett and Muraleedharan 1998), Sri Lanka (Russell and Attenayake 1997) and Zimbabwe (Russell et al. 1997). The selection of these countries for study was based upon four principal criteria:

1. *Low income* – all the countries are low-income countries where capacity tends to be weaker.

2. *Focus on South Asia and Sub-Saharan Africa* – two countries from each of these regions were selected for study. The majority of the world's poor population are clustered in these regions and maintaining some regional focus was desirable to prevent too great a diversity in the culture and bureaucratic tradition of the countries studied.
3. *Common Anglophone and Anglo-colonial heritage* – again this criterion was used to reduce the degree of diversity in the sample and strengthen the ability to generalise to other Anglophone countries in South Asia and Sub-Saharan Africa.
4. *Early and late adjusters* – two of the countries (Sri Lanka and Ghana) are early adjusters which embarked upon structural adjustment and related reforms during the early 1980s; the other two countries (India and Zimbabwe) are late adjusters which embarked upon structural reform during the 1990s.[2] Early and late adjusters were selected partly so that there were differences in the period over which reforms had been implemented, but also because the conditions under which reforms were started and the type of reform programme adopted may vary systematically between early and late adjusters.

The four 'core' country case studies were complemented by less in-depth research and review in Thailand (Bennett et al. 1998), a middle-income country with well-developed state institutions where one might expect New Public Management to be more relevant and more feasible to implement. Thailand is hence termed a 'reference' country, to distinguish it from the 'core' countries.

While the four core country studies were purposively selected to try to reduce the degree of diversity and enhance the ability to generalise to similar countries, there are still clearly considerable differences in the institutions, bureaucratic cultures and traditional cultures of Anglophone countries in the two study regions. Generalising from these four countries to a broader group of low-income countries is hazardous. Furthermore, in India, the analysis focused on Tamil Nadu state simply because within the given time frame and resources, it was not possible to explore the situation more broadly. There is quite a high degree of differentiation between states in India and while Tamil Nadu is not atypical, its health indicators are relatively good compared to other Indian states. Due to these problems of generalisability, application of the study findings to other countries needs to be undertaken with considerable care. Where reliable analyses of the situation in other countries exist, these have been drawn into the discussion in order to support broader applicability of policy conclusions.

In each country, the health sector researchers described and analysed:

- existing organisational arrangements for the provision of health services, and for particular arrangements the relationship between government and service operators;
- the forces sustaining existing service arrangements and the pressures for and resistance to change;
- the performance of existing service arrangements in the provision, production and delivery of public services, with respect to both the adequacy of government's performance of its roles and the efficiency and equity of outcomes;
- factors affecting the capacity of government to undertake its roles.

In order to ensure comparability across country case-studies and at the same time focus the studies in a manageable way, four 'tracer' reforms were selected for study in each country. The tracer reforms selected were:

- bureaucratic commercialisation;
- user fees;
- contracting out services to the private sector;
- enabling and regulating the private sector.

In health care, the relative roles of public and private sectors are commonly analysed according to the part they play in financing health care and in provision of health care (Bennett 1991). These tracer reforms were selected partly to include a mixture of public and private roles in the financing of health care, and public and private roles in the provision of health care. In addition, these reforms reflect the full range of concerns of New Public Management, as set out in Table 1.1. For example, bureaucratic commercialisation focuses on increasing the clarity of goals and purpose of hospital management, while simultaneously strengthening downward accountability. Enabling and regulating the private sector emphasises the creation of stronger incentives for good performance. Finally, these four tracer reforms imply a variety of new roles for the public sector. The relationship between the tracer reforms, the building blocks of NPM, and the new roles implied by the reforms for public and private sectors, are described in Table 1.2.

In addition to the analysis of health sector policy, organisational arrangements and performance, consumer surveys were conducted in each of the core case study countries (Mutizwa-Mangiza 1997, Rakodi 1996 and 1998, Silva, Russell and Rakodi 1997). These studies drew primarily upon a series of focus group discussions, and explored

Table 1.2 Specific reforms studied and relative roles of public and private sectors

Reform of focus	NPM building blocks	Public sector role	Private sector role
Bureaucratic commercial-isation (Autonomous/corporatised hospitals – a form of decentralisation)	*Enhancing responsibility*: ensuring clarity of goals and purpose. *Increasing accountability*: through hospital boards.	Continued public sector financing and provision. New roles: – implement private sector management techniques; – strengthen accountability to community.	No private sector role in financing or provision necessarily required, but the new entity may try to emulate private sector organisations in certain respects, and may draw on private sector skills.
User fees	*Increasing accountability*: facility revenue depends on consumer demand.	Continued public sector provision. New roles: setting fee schedule, organising revenue collection, exemptions, use of revenues.	Private finance.
Contracting out	*Enhancing responsibility*: promote greater transparency through contracts. *Improve performance*: through ensuring link between performance and reward.	Continued public sector financing. New roles: contract with and monitor private sector providers.	Private sector provision of services.
Enabling and regulating the private sector	*Improving performance*: encourage the private sector to expand and offer appropriate quality health care.	Stronger emphasis on regulation plus new approaches. New role: enabling.	Private sector provision and financing.

respondents' attitudes towards public and private sector care and the ongoing reform programmes.

Health was one of four sectors studied as part of a broader programme of research exploring the application of NPM in developing countries. The other sectors examined were water supply, crop marketing and textile promotion.[3] These four sectors were selected as it was thought that the economic characteristics of the services and goods associated with each of the sectors studied were different. In turn, this might imply that the new organisational forms under discussion were more or less appropriate in each of the sectors. The text here draws only to a limited extent upon the findings from the other three sectors.[4]

7.   Structure of the book

Chapters 2 and 3 set the context for consideration of specific reforms. Chapter 2 describes the structure of health systems in each of the study countries and how these systems have performed in terms of improving health outcomes and in terms of various system level indicators. Chapter 3 then attempts to explain performance and provides an overview and interpretation of health sector reform responses. Chapters 4–7 address each of the tracer reforms in turn.

The final two chapters draw together the conclusions emerging from the research. Chapter 8 discusses findings on how capacity issues have affected government performance and the performance of the health sector, and examines the potential of alternative approaches towards capacity building. In Chapter 9 the paradigm of New Public Management, in particular its applicability to the health sectors of developing countries, is reconsidered.

Annex: Market failure arguments

Market failures are considered to stem from:

- consumption characteristics (the extent to which services with characteristics of public goods and externalities are important); and
- production and delivery characteristics (positive and negative externalities, imperfect information of consumers and providers, tendency to monopoly, barriers to entry, economies of scale, scale and risk of investment).

These can be grouped into four types: externalities and public goods, imperfect information, risk and uncertainty, and market structures.

Externalities and public goods

The aspects of market failure which are most commonly cited as grounds for government intervention are the existence of externalities (meaning that the behaviour of one consumer, or producer, affects other parties but this is not taken into account in market transactions) and of public goods (goods whose consumption is non-rival – consumption by one person does not prevent someone else from also consuming, and non-excludable – people cannot be excluded from benefiting). In general, the poorer the quality of the environment and the greater the proportion of infectious and parasitic disease in the total disease profile, the more important are likely to be externality and public goods arguments for state intervention, though these apply most strongly to general public health services rather than to personal health services (with the exception of vaccine-preventable diseases).

Imperfect information

The health sector is typically characterised by uninformed consumers, asymmetry of information between consumers and producers, and producers acting in an agency role for consumers. Consumers have only a limited understanding of what will or will not restore health, or may not even recognise themselves to be ill. The decision not to purchase health care may on occasion lead to irreversible disability or death. Similarly, consumer awareness of the actions required to promote and maintain health (such as hygiene, sanitation, nutrition, antenatal care, vaccination) may be limited amongst a poorly educated population. The producer, on the other hand, has much better information on what the patient requires and usually has considerable influence over what is supplied and consumed. This is of particular concern where the provider benefits financially in proportion to the amount of care provided (as under a fee-for-service payment system).

Risk and uncertainty

The requirement for health care is irregular and unpredictable as it depends upon the incidence of illness. The cost of treatment is also unpredictable and may be very large in relation to income. The market responds to risk and uncertainty by offering insurance. However, the market for health insurance is notably imperfect because of problems of adverse selection and moral hazard.

Market structures

Many market structure characteristics are inherent to medical technology and practice rather than differentiated by country. This applies particularly to the barriers to entry created by the medical profession, and issues of economies of scale, and scale and risk of investment. However, certain market characteristics, such as a tendency to monopoly, will also depend on the degree of development of the private sector.

Apart from the market failure rationale, it is accepted by economists that merit good arguments can be used to justify state intervention for certain types of goods and services which are considered too important to leave to private choice, or where consumers are particularly unable to exercise choice. Health care for children and for the severely mentally ill are cases in point.

2
The Structure and Performance of Health Systems

1. Introduction

The case study countries differed considerably with respect to the structure of their health systems, the roles played by government within these systems, and in terms of health sector performance. This chapter first provides an overview of the primary organisational arrangements for health service delivery, including the relative roles of public and private sectors, and then explores different dimensions of health sector performance. The chapter aims to provide readers with an understanding of how the health systems of the study countries operated and what these systems had achieved.

The discussion of organisational arrangements does not describe in detail any particular arrangement, but rather provides an overview of how the various health systems in the study countries operated. More detailed information on specific operational arrangements is given in Chapters 4–7.

Monitoring performance was not a principal aim of the study. Consequently no primary data on performance were collected; instead, researchers relied upon existing data sources, and occasionally this created problems in terms of the reliability or comparability of data. Both the performance of the sector as a whole and the performance of government within the health sector are discussed here. A complex relationship exists between these two dimensions. To a certain extent a strong government capacity to perform, combined with an appropriate role for government, is likely to contribute to strong performance of the sector as a whole. However, the roles of government are diverse (including regulating, policy-making and direct provision) and government may perform some of these roles better than others. For example, weak performance by government with respect to direct service provision may have limited impact upon the overall performance of the sector if much of the provision occurs in the private sector and government plays an effective role in terms of regulation and broad policies.

The first section on performance explores intermediate system-level results, specifically relating to technical objectives (quality, equity, efficiency and sustainability). The discussion of system level indicators encompasses both input indicators (such as staff availability), process indicators (such as accessibility and prescription patterns) and output indicators (such as utilisation data). As much of the data about performance relate to the public health sector only, a separate section devoted to performance of the private health sector is included, as is a section on bureaucratic performance. The second section on performance considers outcomes of the health sector (and social and economic processes more broadly), considering changes in the population's health in the case study countries. Interpretation of these data requires broader background information about demographic and socio-economic con-text; this is covered in more depth in Chapter 3.

2.   Organisational arrangements for service provision

The main organisational arrangements for service provision were briefly discussed in Chapter 1, where a distinction was drawn between public and private roles in the financing of health care, and public and private roles in the provision of health care. Using this form of categorisation, four main types of organisational arrangement can be identified:

1. public financing and provision: government both funds health care and adopts direct roles of service management and delivery;
2. public financing and private provision: government funds health care, but adopts an indirect role of service provision by arranging contracts or subsidising private providers in a more informal way;
3. private financing and public provision: private agents including users finance health care services which are delivered by publicly owned agents;
4. private financing and provision: the government role is confined to regulation and standard setting; services are both financed and provided by private sector agents.

In all countries, both core and reference, the predominant arrange-ments were the first (public funding and provision) and the fourth (private funding and provision). In terms of public funding and provision, organisational arrangements were in general similar across the countries. The Ministry of Health (MOH) was at the apex of a pyramid, with lower management levels below it, and a structure of services – at least in theory – consisting of peripheral outpatient facilities, local hospitals, general hospitals, and central hospitals with referral and supervisory relationships between them. Some specific features differed: for example, in some countries local government authorities had some role in the provision of services (especially municipalities in India, and to a lesser extent elsewhere), though in none of the countries did local government have prime responsibility for health. India differed in its federal structure, which separated government health functions between the federal and state level, with the state level taking prime responsibility for the provision of health services. Countries also differed in the degree of decentralisation of management responsibilities within the hierarchical public system, and the extent to which the MOH engaged in management itself or restricted its role to policy, planning and regulation.

Pure private arrangements (private funding and provision) can be sub-classified by whether the services are for-profit or not-for-profit; draw on allopathic or traditional systems of medicine; and provide ambulatory or inpatient care. Here there was greater variation between countries on all these dimensions. The strong church presence in health services in the two African countries was not replicated elsewhere, though India did have strong non-governmental organisations (NGOs), often indigenous ones. Thus Ghana, Zimbabwe and India all had a substantial number of not-for-profit suppliers of health care, with Sri Lanka being the exception, probably because the government had been very proactive in the provision of health care. Both India and Sri Lanka had a strong indigenous system of medicine (Ayurveda). The nature of the care provided by the formal 'modern' (allopathic) private sector depended substantially on its degree of development. Ghana had the least developed private sector, in which ambulatory care dominated. The other countries all had a substantial network of both ambulatory and inpatient facilities, though concentrated in large urban centres. Although data are scarce, it seems likely that only in India, Sri Lanka and Thailand did private allopathic providers market their services to the bulk of the population, with different segments of the private market serving different socio-economic groups and private medical practitioners operating even in urban slums. However, this latter market was primarily for outpatient care, since hospitalisation was far more expensive. In Ghana and Zimbabwe, the poor were unable to afford the fees of the formal private sector, and instead patronised informal and traditional practitioners.

The extent of the mixed organisational arrangement, involving public funding and private provision, was extremely limited. In theory, private provision could be subdivided into a situation where assets remained in public ownership but were managed by private operators, and where provision was entirely private. In practice, it was rare for the public sector to bring in private management to health facilities: the preferred arrangement was to contract out services to private providers, though even these arrangements were relatively few, as Chapter 6 shows. There was also a range of less formal subsidies to the private sector, which Chapter 7 examines. The only significant flow of funds between public and private sectors was in Ghana and Zimbabwe, where government provided substantial subsidies to church providers. This resulted in a perception that they were 'quasi-public' rather than private providers. In Thailand, the civil servants medical benefit scheme gave access to private hospital care[1] and the compulsory social health insurance scheme allowed a choice between public and private hospitals. Subsidies in the form of tax exemptions to the private health sector in Zimbabwe, India and Thailand may have been substantial, but data on them were not readily available.

A more difficult to classify arrangement between public and private sectors is where essentially the same body of doctors work in both sectors. In Zimbabwe, Sri Lanka, Thailand and some states in India this was legally allowed; in Ghana only locums were permitted, but in countries and states where it is not legally allowed it is usually none the less common. While this does not change the formal pattern of financing and ownership, it substantially affects the interaction of the two sectors and means that sectors which are formally quite separate, in practice interact.

All countries had a framework of rules and regulations which applied to the private sector, and is considered in depth in Chapter 7.

3.   Performance

A critical issue in terms of assessing performance is the standards or goals against which performance should be judged. There is considerable consensus on the technical criteria (generally specified as quality, equity, efficiency and sustainability, or some variation thereof). However, there may be difficult trade-offs between them. The most commonly cited trade-off is that between equity and efficiency. Hence it may become necessary to assess performance against government's own policy objectives: was the government striving to improve equity and provide access to all, or was it more concerned with sustainability or efficiency?

This raises a further complicating factor in assessing performance, namely the fact that stated 'formal' policy objectives may differ from informal or unofficial goals. Because of the difficulty of identifying unofficial objectives, it was not feasible in the case studies to attempt to assess performance against them. None the less, where it is likely that formal and informal goals were incongruent (or competing), this is considered in the analysis as an explanatory factor.

During the past 5–10 years, there has been substantial interest in developing systems of performance indicators to track the effects of health policy development and implementation within countries and to allow international comparisons of performance (Knowles 1997, McPake and Kutzin 1997). The approach used here draws from these sources.

3.1 System level results

Quality

It is common to break down an assessment of quality of care into input, process and outcome indicators. While data on inputs were quite readily available, hard evidence on both process and outcome aspects of quality was much more patchy. Consequently, this section primarily uses input data and draws upon more anecdotal evidence about other aspects of quality where available. In addition, substantial use is made of the series of consumer surveys conducted for the research programme which provided consumer perspectives on quality of care.

Input indicators (see Table 2.1) suggested that there was quite different resource availability between the different study countries. In India there was a remarkably high physician:population ratio. Many Indians saw medical training as a way to guarantee both status and income. Private medical schools had grown rapidly to respond to this demand, and there had been a considerable increase in the number of trained physicians. Despite this, many vacancies in the public sector persisted as doctors

Table 2.1 Input indicators for health services

	Ghana	Zimbabwe	India	Sri Lanka	Thailand
Total no. physicians per 1,000 people	0.077 (1995)	0.135 (1990)	0.407 (1993)	0.146 (1993)	0.233 (1992)
Total no. hospital beds per 1,000 people	1.46 (1990)	0.51 (1990)	0.79 (1991)	2.74 (1990)	1.71 (1992)

Source: World Development Indicators, 1998.
The year the data relate to is shown in parenthesis.

commonly preferred to work privately. Sri Lanka appeared to have a relatively high number of hospital beds per head of the population. Thailand seemed relatively better endowed than most of the core countries studied with respect to both physicians and hospital beds. The two African countries (particularly Ghana) were much less well endowed with physicians, although Ghana had a relatively high number of hospital beds.

In the core countries, there was striking similarity in the conclusions drawn by the researchers about quality of care. In terms of structural aspects, government health services, especially in rural areas, were commonly observed to suffer from:

- shortages of drugs and supplies;
- staffing shortages and inappropriate staff mix;
- poorly maintained machinery and buildings.

There was also considerable agreement about problems associated with process aspects of care, including:

- long waiting times;
- poor staff attitudes;
- the limited range of services available at the peripheral level;
- inappropriate (too short) opening hours.

None the less, while there was considerable consensus about the range and severity of problems of quality of care amongst government health providers, there was also some agreement that the technical quality of care in some government facilities was higher than that in any private facility.

One concern about quality of care which differed between the African and South Asian countries related to government physicians' private practice. In both India and Sri Lanka, nearly all government doctors also carried out private practice. In India it was commonplace for government doctors to neglect their public sector responsibilities in favour of their private practices: doctors spent very few hours in government facilities, and were believed to channel some of their public clients into their private practice. In Sri Lanka, doctors could operate private clinics only outside regular working hours but there were concerns about 'leakage' of government drugs and supplies into the private sector. In Zimbabwe a similar set of problems had arisen, but only during the 1990s when dwindling government budgets and deteriorating salary and benefit packages had led many physicians to neglect their public duties in favour of private practice. There was increasing concern about the impact of this upon training of new physicians in Zimbabwe (Mutizwa-Mangiza 1998). In Ghana the formal private sector was smaller, and this perhaps made the problem less severe.

While staffing shortages were a concern across all types of public health facility in Zimbabwe, in Sri Lanka and India they were restricted to certain types of facility. In particular it was difficult to find qualified staff willing to work in the rural areas and at lower-level facilities (such as primary health care facilities in India). This contributed to poor quality care in these facilities. While staff shortages at higher level and urban facilities in India were not problematic, the very poor motivation of staff working in virtually all government facilities was of major concern.

One potential indicator of poor quality is low utilisation rates. In Ghana, there were only about 0.3 consultations per capita per annum in government facilities compared to about 2.0 in Tanzania and Uganda. Data from Sri Lanka also suggested low utilisation (about 0.2 consultations per capita in government facilities), but the presence of a large private primary care sector is likely to be a significant explanatory factor.

Consumer perceptions of quality of care

Focus group discussions conducted with the general population in each of the study countries described how consumers perceived the quality of care provided by public and private health care providers (see Table 2.2) (Mutizwa-Mangiza 1997, Rakodi 1996 and 1998, Silva, Russell and Rakodi 1997).

In general, the perception of consumers about quality of care supported the descriptions given above. The types of criticisms formulated by consumers were similar, but there were some clear differences between the countries in consumers' overall perception of public sector health care quality. In Sri Lanka, for example, despite specific criticisms made about waiting times, the brevity of consultations, drug shortages and over-crowding in hospitals, respondents were, by and large, satisfied with the care received in government facilities. The same cannot be said of Indian respondents. While the respondents in Tamil Nadu state valued the services provided by the front-line Village Health Nurses (particularly maternal and child health and ante-natal care), they were highly critical of services provided at Primary Health Centres and hospitals, and felt that these services had declined significantly over the past decade. In Zimbabwe, there were criticisms of services but many of these, such as drug shortages, linen shortages, fewer investigations due to broken equipment and inadequate food in hospitals, were due primarily to lack of

Table 2.2 Strengths and weaknesses of care provided in government facilities: consumer perspectives

Ghana	Zimbabwe	India	Sri Lanka
Strengths			
Good antenatal care, family planning and child health services	Effective antenatal, maternity care, and well-baby clinics	Effective family planning services. Good ante-natal and child health advice provided by Village Health Nurse	Good maternity services
Cheaper than private facilities	Cheaper than private facilities		Free or cheaper than private facilities
Better equipped than private	Clean and tidy (municipal services)		Many facilities and all equipment
Well-qualified and more skilled staff	More comprehensive and effective treatment than private sector		Faith in staff
			Provide emergency care
Weaknesses			
Slow service	Long queues and slow service, even for emergency cases	Lack of available staff – staff in private practice	Long queues
Poor staff motivation, some problems of poor interpersonal skills	Poorly motivated and abusive staff	Poor interpersonal skills: impolite, careless	Poor staff attitudes
Dirty facilities, bad smells	Overcrowded wards, shortages of linen at some facilities	Lack of cleanliness	Overcrowded wards and lack of cleanliness
Drug shortages	Drug shortages	Drug shortages	Drug shortages
Need to pay tips, even sometimes for indigent or emergency cases	Fewer investigations due to breakdown of equipment and shortage of supplies	Costly due to bribes	
	Lack of available physicians in some facilities due to private practice	Poor diagnosis and treatment – overhasty and careless	Limited consultation time with patients
	Small amounts and poor quality food	Use of improperly sterilised needles	
	Discriminatory attitudes to exempted patients	Discriminatory attitudes to low castes	

Sources: Mutizwa-Mangiza 1997, Rakodi 1996 and 1998, Silva, Russell and Rakodi 1997.

resources in government budgets. The overriding concern of respondents appeared to be that government health care charges had made care unaffordable. Public sector health care facilities were the preferred option for serious conditions:

> Private doctors and hospitals are okay for minor illnesses, but when one is very ill it is better to go to a government hospital where many doctors can look after you. (Mutizwa-Mangiza 1997: 19)

Respondents in Ghana also appreciated the better clinical skills of public sector staff and the greater availability of equipment in public facilities (although such equipment was not always working). As elsewhere, there were criticisms of unhygienic conditions, drug availability and health worker motivation, but fewer complaints about hurried or careless treatment. Ghanaian respondents seemed to accept the necessity to pay tips to public sector health staff and even commented that this had improved quality, but cases were resented where indigent or emergency patients were denied care due to their inability to tip.

Although for typical illnesses the choice between public and private provider was finely balanced or in favour of the private sector, for most maternal and child health and family planning services, the public sector was recognised to offer superior care in virtually all respects in all countries.

Health expenditure and financial sustainability

Data on health expenditure were often inconsistent, reflecting the fact that most developing countries do not have well-established procedures to track health expenditures. The data in Table 2.3 were taken from the World Development Indicators and World Bank (1993). They give an approximate picture of the overall significance of health spending in the economy, how health financing is split between public and private sectors, and the role of donors in supporting health finance.

While Sri Lanka demonstrated impressive health indicators, as shown later in this chapter, it devoted a relatively small share of its total GDP to health care. However, the majority of expenditure (approximately 75 per cent) took place in the public sector. In contrast, India and Zimbabwe both had relatively high proportions of GDP devoted to health care, but a much larger proportion of expenditure (approximately 65 per cent in Zimbabwe and 78 per cent in India) was private. The share of private spending in Ghana appears extremely low: it is likely that payments to traditional practitioners and the informal sector (such as drug sellers),

Table 2.3   Health expenditure patterns

	Ghana	Zimbabwe	India	Sri Lanka	Thailand
Health expenditure private as % GDP	0.09 (1995)	4.20 (1991)	4.38 (1991)	0.44 (1993)	3.88 (1992)
Health expenditure public as % GDP	1.35 (1995)	2.27 (1991)	1.22 (1991)	1.42 (1994)	1.32 (1992)
Total health expenditure as % GDP	1.44 (1995)	6.47 (1991)	5.6 (1991)	1.88 (1993)	5.25 (1992)
Health expenditure per capita $	14 (1990)	42 (1990)	21 (1990)	18 (1990)	73 (1990)
Aid as % of total health expenditure	14.2 (1990)	10.0 (1990)	1.6 (1990)	7.4 (1990)	0.9 (1990)

Source: World Development Indicators 1998, World Bank, 1993.
The year the data relate to is shown in parenthesis.

who accounted for much of the Ghanaian private sector, were under-reported.

Health expenditure per capita was considerably higher in Thailand than in the core countries. Zimbabwe, however was something of an outlier, per capita spending on health care being more than twice that in any of the other core countries.

Particularly in the African core countries, donor funding accounted for a considerable proportion of health sector expenditure, raising concerns about sustainability. Another potential indicator of the sustainability of the public health sector (as well as of the government's commitment to health) is the percentage of the government budget allocated to health. In Zimbabwe government health spending was quite high at the beginning of the 1990s (approximately 6.8 per cent of total government spending in 1990/91) and increased to 8.0 per cent in 1996/97. However, despite this increasing share of government funds, real government allocations to health had declined because of the economic recession and the consequent reduction in the total government budget. In India a complex pattern of central government and state government allocations to health care complicated analyses. However, there had been persistent criticism (Duggal 1997) of the level of government allocations to health care, and in general these allocations had declined since the mid-1980s. For example, in 1985/6 health expenditure constituted 3.29 per cent of total central government expenditure, but by 1994/95 this had declined to 2.63 per cent. Health expenditure in Thailand during the 1980s accounted for approximately 11–12 per cent of total government expenditure, and this ratio had been fairly constant.

Equity

Public health care systems are frequently criticised for being inequitable, focusing resources upon more affluent urban populations (World Bank 1987). Commonly this is associated with a bias towards high-cost hospital services, rather than primary care. While distribution across population types and service types are logically separate (the former concerning questions of equity, and the latter concerning questions of allocative efficiency) they are so highly correlated that they are addressed jointly here.

In Zimbabwe during the period immediately post-Independence, much was done to correct the urban and curative bias of the colonial health system. However, a considerable bias to curative care still existed with the eight largest hospitals in urban areas consuming over 50 per cent of recurrent resources (Table 2.4). In Ghana the available data consistently showed that government services disproportionately served urban populations and higher-income households. For example, nearly two-thirds of MOH doctors were based at the two teaching hospitals. In consequence, nearly 90 per cent of consultations in Accra were with medical doctors, compared to 28 per cent in the rural savannah areas. By the end of the 1980s, primary health care in Ghana still received only about 20–25 per cent of the total MOH budget.

Sri Lanka had probably a better record than the other core countries in allocating resources to primary care and rural areas, but it still had a significant urban and tertiary service bias. The format of budgets made it difficult to analyse allocations across different levels of service, but 1994 data suggested that approximately 38.5 per cent of total government health care expenditure went to tertiary and specialist hospitals. The distribution of government resources in India gave surprising emphasis to preventive and promotive services: in 1990/1, of the total state and central

Table 2.4   Recurrent resource allocation by service level in Zimbabwe

	% total allocation
Central hospitals (N = 4)	33.26
General hospitals (N = 4)	17.33
Provincial hospitals (N = 8)	12.47
District and rural hospitals, health centres	36.94

Source: Cripps, 1997.

level health budget, approximately 30 per cent went to preventive and promotive services, 47 per cent to curative care and health facility operations and the remainder was spent on research, training and capital investment (World Bank 1994). Although compared to other countries the Indian government budget appeared to be biased towards preventive services, it should be borne in mind that the government contributed a very small percentage of total health spending.

During the 1980s the Thai government made a concerted effort to shift resources to remote rural areas, and with some success. Spending in rural areas increased from 47.6 per cent of the MOH budget in 1979 to 52.2 per cent in 1990. Like the core countries studied, Thailand had also had difficulty in shifting resources to lower levels of the health care system and to primary and promotive services. In 1990 only about 30 per cent of the MOH budget went to the lowest levels of the health care system, i.e. district and *tambon* health services, and analysis of the budget by activity showed that only 25 per cent of the total MOH budget went to preventive and promotive activities.

Data on service accessibility were very approximate. In Sri Lanka every village had a free (government) health care facility within 5 km. In contrast, in India only about 35 per cent of the total population had health centres within 2 km of their place of residence. In Ghana only about 50 per cent of the population had 'access' to health facilities.

Several of the country case studies conducted suggested that user fees had exacerbated problems of inequity in access to health care. This evidence is considered separately in Chapter 5.

Efficiency

Efficiency is commonly broken down into its allocative and technical components. Several aspects of allocative efficiency were addressed in the previous paragraphs. For example, the discussion of equity noted a bias in resource allocation towards higher levels of the health system, and towards urban areas. These biases are not only inequitable but also contribute to allocative inefficiency: it would be more efficient to use resources at those points where they would most likely have greater impact.

Technical efficiency in the health sector is difficult to explore in a rigorous manner because of differences in quality of care: while it is straightforward to show relative differences in the costs of providing care, this does not necessarily imply that the lower cost provider is more efficient since difficult-to-measure differences in quality of care may contribute to observed cost differentials. In several of the countries studied, similar health care units were observed to have quite different unit cost patterns, but it was unclear whether these were due to differences in efficiency. Similarly, although some sparse data were available comparing costs in public and private health care facilities, these generally were not able to derive firm conclusions about relative efficiency of facilities in different types of ownership. Hence the analysis here of technical efficiency relies upon proxy indicators, and observations of how health care facilities produced services.

One of the key concerns in each of the core countries was that patients tended to bypass low-level facilities, which they perceived to offer substandard quality of care, in favour of higher-level facilities. As a consequence, there was simultaneously overcrowding at the higher levels of the health system and underutilisation of lower level facilities. For example, in Zimbabwe, bed occupancy rates (BOR) in government district hospitals were less than 50 per cent while the central hospitals had occupancy rates in excess of 100 per cent. Data from Sri Lanka were similar: average BOR in rural hospitals in 1994 was 50 per cent compared to 103 per cent in provincial hospitals. A study in Ghana concluded that there was excess hospital capacity in many areas, with BOR in government hospitals in the range of 35–50 per cent. This was due to inappropriate specialty mixes in these hospitals combined with poor geographical distribution (McNaught and Lazarus 1994).

Inefficiencies in government facilities also arose due to poor human resource management. For example, in Ghana it was found that payroll expenditure per hospital bed in the public sector was more than double that in mission hospitals, while non-personnel recurrent expenditure per bed was less than half the mission hospital average (Smithson 1993). Testing of an early set of staffing norms (for all staff excluding nurses) indicated that current staffing profiles exceeded required staffing by about 129 per cent.

In India it was widely recognised that government employed an unnecessarily high number of unskilled staff in its health facilities. Government policies which had attempted to create jobs, particularly for disadvantaged groups, had contributed to this inefficiency. Data from Sri Lanka showed that private hospitals used far fewer physicians than government hospitals; however, the implications of this for quality of care were unclear (Alailima and Mohideen 1984). A further staffing problem in India was that remote primary health centres were unable to fill many posts whereas facilities in urban areas were often overstaffed. One estimate indicated that recently constructed primary health centres in remote areas had only 59 per cent of the norm of posts filled, compared to higher level community health centres which had 142 per cent of the norm of posts filled.

In Ghana, Zimbabwe and India, the limited contribution of public finance to health care had become a major problem. Governments had established an extensive network of health facilities, but the funding available for complementary inputs such as drugs, supplies and maintenance was too low for these facilities to operate properly.

The country studies in Zimbabwe, India and Ghana each noted problems of inefficient drug use in the public sector. In Ghana, the problems were said to include an excessive number of prescriptions, and unnecessary use of antibiotics and injections. In India and Zimbabwe there were shortages of key drugs (in India shortages of curative medicines were particularly acute) which prevented other inputs from being effective.

While Thailand experienced some similar problems (for example, bypassing of primary care facilities and inefficient staff mix) the nature of inefficiency was substantially different. In particular the absolute lack of funds was much less of a problem, and there were more concerns about inefficiencies springing from the inappropriate use of high technology equipment and the overprovision of services.

Private health sector performance

All the core country studies observed that the inadequate quality of care in government facilities had forced many consumers to seek services in the private sector. Participants in the focus group discussions were clear as to the benefits of private sector health care providers (Mutizwa-Mangiza 1997, Rakodi 1996, 1998; Silva, Russell and Rakodi 1997). They were universally perceived to offer:

- a faster service;
- a more convenient service in terms of opening hours;
- better staff attitudes;
- longer consultations and more individual attention.

However, despite these positive impressions, there was also some caution on the part of the general population about the use of private providers. Awareness of the problems most commonly associated with private practice seemed most limited in India. There, while respondents acknowledged that private practitioners may overprescribe, this seemed a very minor concern compared to the hazards of seeking public sector care.

In Ghana, Zimbabwe and Sri Lanka, concerns about private care were more extensive and more sophisticated. In Sri Lanka it was recognised that private providers often had limited facilities, that they lacked good referral links with other facilities, that they often put excessive emphasis upon (income-generating) diagnostic tests, and that they were expensive. Zimbabwean respondents were quite hostile to private facilities, particularly for serious conditions. They were particularly sceptical of the motivation of private practitioners, and suggested that they did not necessarily care for people, but simply wanted their money.

There was little hard empirical evidence either to support or refute respondents' assertions about quality of care in the private sector. In India, both internal analysts and external observers agreed that the quality of private sector care left much to be desired, and unethical practices were widespread. Data from Thailand on quality of care in a small sample of public and private hospitals found complex differences in how hospitals functioned, but it was difficult to find any clear pattern in terms of objective measures of quality of care (Tangcharoensathien 1996). Broader issues about the scale, scope and nature of the private health care sector are discussed in more depth in Chapter 7.

Bureaucratic performance

In some of the countries studied, such as Thailand, there had always been a kudos and high status associated with being a member of the bureaucracy. In India such a mystique existed around the elite bureaucrats (Indian Administrative Services, IAS) but was not true more broadly of civil servants. To what extent was this reputation deserved? This section moves away from government performance with respect to service delivery, towards a consideration of the performance of bureaucratic functions. A surprisingly similar array of problems and issues emerged from the country case studies.

In each country there was perceived to be an excessively centralised decision-making process. The Ghanaian health sector, during the past few years, had attempted to address this problem, but the issue of over-centralisation was so deeply embedded in the management style of the broader public sector that it was difficult and slow to overcome. In both Sri Lanka and Zimbabwe, it was observed that overcentralisation of decision-making meant that central government was too overwhelmed by operational management and fire fighting for it to fulfil its strategic roles effectively. Issues of overcentralisation were particularly difficult in India, where state–central government relations added further complexities to the centralisation issue.

Overcentralisation was often associated with vertical programmes. For example, in Ghana until recently, the central MOH was structured around heads of different cadres (such as Chief Nursing Officer) and heads of different vertical programmes. Recent reforms in Ghana have changed this to provide a more integrated approach. In India virtually all priority services (such as malaria control, family planning, AIDS control) were delivered through largely vertical programmes, over which the central government had great authority.

Management systems (planning, budgeting, human resource management, finance and information systems) were viewed to be weak in all the core countries, with very limited strategic planning taking place. Even in Sri Lanka where it was recognised that MOH plans were competently compiled, it was observed that they tended to be unambitious, they failed to address more complex problems (such as labour indiscipline and pilfering) and they totally excluded the private sector. This was also largely true of the five-year plans developed by the Health Ministry in Thailand. In India until recently, plans emphasised the achievement of output targets (such as the number of family planning acceptors, or cases of TB treated). This focus upon quantitative targets frequently distorted health worker incentives and led to some perverse outcomes. In recent years the government had moved away from this system. Whilst a health sector planning capacity existed at the central level in India, there had been no health planning units at the state level until recently, when units had been set up primarily in those states where the World Bank had been active.

Budgeting systems were largely historical, with only limited efforts to rationalise and prioritise resource allocations. In India, the mix of state and federal financing for health care created over-complex and unmanageable financing systems. Furthermore, in India (and to a lesser extent in other countries) bureaucratic systems focused upon control (by the centre) rather than enabling local level action. This control focus meant that bureaucratic rules, particularly relating to budgetary and financial systems, were commonly very cumbersome. Whilst there were continuing attempts in all four core countries to strengthen bureaucratic performance within the health sector, these efforts seemed most far advanced in Ghana.

In terms of broader aspects of bureaucratic performance, in both India and Sri Lanka the problems associated with political interference in bureaucratic processes were acknowledged. Furthermore, bureaucratic performance in India was marred by corruption throughout all sectors of government, which meant that most of the population mistrusted the public sector to a significant degree.

3.2 Results in terms of change in health status

Table 2.5 highlights the very impressive achievements in health status made in Sri Lanka compared to the other core countries, exceeding even those of Thailand in some respects. The data given for India in the table is for the country as a whole, and this masks very substantial differences in health outcomes between states. Life expectancy at birth in Zimbabwe was surprisingly low, particularly compared to the relatively low infant mortality rate, and is likely to have been due to the increasing burden of AIDS in that country.

Taking an historical perspective on health status also provides interesting results (see Figure 2.1). Sri Lanka had demonstrated good health status indicators since the early 1970s, but had managed to improve them further. India, which had started the 1970s with by far the highest IMR of any of the core countries, had reduced infant mortality rates nearly by half. Progress in the two African countries had been a lot slower, and in Zimbabwe had particularly slackened during the 1990s. During the post-Independence period, Zimbabwe had made significant improvements in health status (as indicated by measures of life expectancy, infant mortality and maternal mortality) through redressing inequalities in the sector and expanding coverage of basic services. However, it had not been possible to sustain this record:

> The relatively favourable picture of improving health in Zimbabwe did not last into the 1990s. ... By the end of that decade [1980s], slippage was clearly evident. ... At the same time large numbers of health professionals began leaving Government service and even leaving Zimbabwe. The number of nurses per capita fell by 17% between 1988 and 1993. (UNICEF 1994).

Table 2.5   Health outcomes

	Ghana	Zimbabwe	India	Sri Lanka	Thailand
Life expectancy at birth (total)	58.9	56.2	62.7	72.8	69.1
Infant mortality rate	71.02	56.08	65.32	15.35	34.12
<5 years mortality rate	110	86	85	19	38
Measles immunisation % children <1	49	77	84	84	86
Total fertility rate	5.02	3.90	3.14	2.25	1.78

Source: World Development Indicators, 1998.

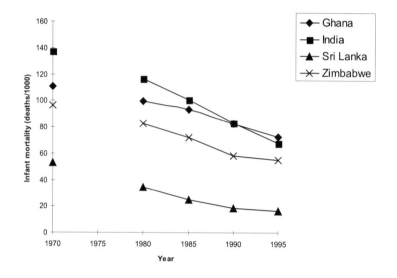

Figure 2.1   Trends in infant mortality, 1970–95
Source: World Bank Indicators, 1998.

UNICEF attributed this decline in health status to deterioration of health sector performance, as well as the macro-economic situation in Zimbabwe.

Given the influence of level of income on health status, it is helpful to standardise for income in these comparisons. Figure 2.2, using data from the 1999 World Health Report (WHO 1999), compares the actual IMR and female life expectancy (FLE) to the level that would be predicted given a country's income level, for four different time periods. The indicator represents the percentage difference between observed and expected: in the case of IMR, a negative number indicates better performance, and in the case of FLE a negative number represents a worse performance.[2]

The graphs emphasise the consistency in the relative performance of the countries over time, as well as the markedly better performance of Sri Lanka and the markedly worse performance of India. Ghana performs rather close to the mean, and Zimbabwe shows a marked worsening of performance in the most recent time period. The much higher performance in Sri Lanka has often been used to argue that governments can take actions which deliver better health status than that predicted by their level of GNP. In Sri Lanka it is commonly said that focusing upon primary health care and female literacy have been key in delivering these

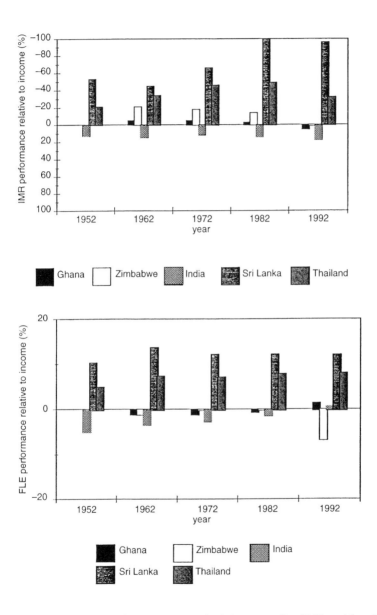

Figure 2.2 Performance relative to income for infant mortality (IMR) and female
life expectancy (FLE)
Source: WHO, 1999.

impressive results. Lower levels of absolute poverty may also have been a factor.

Given the multiple determinants of health status, it is impossible to relate closely health sector performance and health outcomes. Health sector performance is clearly just one amongst many influences upon health status, and is generally thought to be one of the less significant determinants. Overall economic performance and related government policies are likely to play an important role, as the situation in Zimbabwe suggested, not just because they directly affect people's welfare but also because they affect the volume of resources available for health and related sectors such as education and public infrastructure for water and sanitation. Chapter 3 explores in more detail the macro-economic context and how it affected health outcomes and health policy in the study countries.

4.   Conclusions

In broad terms there was considerable similarity in the structure of the health provision arrangements in all five study countries: a network of publicly financed and provided services coexisted with privately financed and provided services. Public financing of private services was observed only to a limited degree, and with the exception of Thailand, public services were largely financed from the public purse. Despite these gross similarities the relative sizes of public and private sectors, and the overall performance of the health sector, differed considerably.

In terms of health sector performance, Sri Lanka performed best in terms of both overall health outcomes and government performance (as measured by indicators of quality of care in government facilities). India had consistently underfunded public health care services with resulting problems of resource availability. Moreover, bureaucratic problems in India (such as overcentralisation) contributed to the poor performance of the health sector. Performance in the two Sub-Saharan African countries had deteriorated considerably in recent years, particularly in Zimbabwe, which once had a relatively highly performing health sector. Much of this deterioration can be linked to the macro-economic crisis which had affected all sectors of the economy.

Differences emerged between countries in the relative roles of public and private sectors. India and Zimbabwe spent a larger proportion of GNP on health care than the other two core countries, but a substantial proportion of this was associated with expenditure in the private sector. In contrast, a rather higher proportion of health expenditure in Ghana and

Sri Lanka was public, but overall a lesser share of GNP was spent on health. Given the relatively poor performance of the health sector in India and Zimbabwe there seemed to be some grounds for questioning the effectiveness of private health sector expenditure.

As the four core countries were selected with the aim of drawing conclusions for a broader group of low income countries, it is worthwhile considering how representative they are of the regions in which they are situated. The two Sub-Saharan African countries appear to be fairly typical, although Zimbabwe was clearly more affluent than many other African countries and has a considerably larger formal private health sector than commonly found in Africa. Sri Lanka possessed better health indicators than other South Asian countries, though factors outside the health sector rather than the health sector itself were important influences. Thus although the Sri Lankan health system may have performed better than other systems within the region, it does not appear to be a complete outlier.

3
Explanations of Performance and Reform Responses

1. Introduction

This chapter provides an overview of health sector reform in the five study countries. The policy context, content and process are each analysed (Walt and Gilson 1994). New Institutional Economics emphasises that most institutional change is incremental and slow and hence the historical structure of institutions will affect the speed and success of reform. Accordingly, the following section on context explores in some detail the historical development of the health system in the study countries. The contextual section also addresses macro-economic and social issues, describing trends in economic and social indicators and the design and implementation of structural adjustment programmes. Consideration of these broader contextual issues helps explain the health system performance described in the previous chapter.

Subsequent sections of this chapter describe and analyse the current contents of the health sector reform agendas and the processes through which reform agendas were constructed. The final section explores the relevance of alternative theoretical frameworks to explaining existing patterns of state intervention and proposed reforms.

2. Contextual factors

2.1 Historical development of the health system

All four core countries had in common a history of colonisation by Great Britain (in contrast, Thailand had never been colonised). They followed a general pattern that Western health services had been introduced by the colonial power, initially to cater for the needs of the military, civil service and settler communities (Zwi and Mills 1995). However, given the prevalence of communicable diseases, protecting expatriates meant that disease in the indigenous population had also to be addressed, and in some areas, ensuring a workforce healthy enough to work productively in plantations and mines was a consideration, though sometimes a weak one because of the ready supply of unskilled labour (Packard 1990). Epidemics in the late nineteenth and early twentieth centuries encouraged the extension of colonial influence, and at a time when there was greater confidence in the ability of medical science to conquer disease (Arnold 1988).

Amongst the four core countries, a number of common themes emerge in terms of health system development, namely: a central role for the state in health service provision, a strong bias towards curative and hospital services, and the development of powerful constituencies within the health sector. Interestingly, while each country after independence at least formally espoused a strong state role in health, attitudes towards the development of a private health sector varied between countries. Each of these themes is considered next.

A strong state role

The very limited existence of private practice and charitable activities in tropical colonies meant a greater role for the state, though hampered by lack of resources. It was not until after the First World War that there was significant expansion of state medical services in the tropical colonies, and even then outreach was very limited. However, a close relationship had been established between state power and Western medicine: Arnold (1988) argues that in the colonies of Africa, Asia and the Pacific, medicine was one of the most intrusive expressions of state power.

In Ghana health provision had long been seen as a legitimate and necessary role of government. From the patriarchal outlook of the colonial government, through the planned development and modernisation of the Nkrumah era and the authoritarian regimes of the 1960s and 1970s to the present day, health and health services have traditionally been regarded as a responsibility of the state. Private financing and provision were not banned, but neither were they encouraged or regarded as the dominant agents of health sector development. In Zimbabwe a strong state role in health has been emphasised from independence, and is heavily rooted in the political ideology of socialism.

Western medicine was brought to India by the colonisers to protect the health of the army and the European community. Indeed Ramasubban (1982) argues that the protection of the army and the European civilian population was at all times the highest priority of colonial health policy for British India in the nineteenth century. There were regular epidemics before the First World War, but it was the perceived threat to the health of British troops that first provided the impetus for sanitary reform and the beginnings of a public health administration (Arnold 1988).

A proactive role for government in health care was given even greater importance after independence. The All India Bhore Committee Report (1946) had emphasised that the state should take responsibility for providing health care, and that this should be accessible irrespective of ability to pay. The emphasis upon a strong state role was of course consistent with overall development policy, which until recently gave a prime role to the state not merely in setting policy but also in service delivery over a wide range of sectors. Similar developments had occurred at the state level; for example, the introduction of the Public Health Act in 1939 in Madras conferred on the government wide-ranging power to protect the health of the people.

However, a marked feature of Indian health development, in contrast to other countries studied, is that this aim had never been matched by anything near the level of resources needed to achieve it, and health has never had the share of the government budget achieved elsewhere.

In Sri Lanka public demands for state action in health care occurred prior to Independence, as a result of the introduction in 1931 of an elected assembly with universal franchise. Health care rapidly came to be perceived as a basic right for all citizens, and this was embodied in the constitution, which required that every citizen had access to adequate health services.

The partial exception to the central role for government which emerged in all four of the core countries was the special situation of mission health facilities, particularly in Sub-Saharan Africa. Missionaries entered with the colonisers,[1] and introduced medical care both as a part of proselytising activities and also from a genuine concern for the welfare of the colonised. In Zimbabwe missions were the first European institutions to provide medical care to the rural populations outside the settler areas, which were of low priority to the settler regime (Government of the Republic of Zimbabwe 1981), and were still by far the dominant provider in these areas at Independence. In India, church organisations were also important in hospital development.

The four core countries therefore all demonstrated a history of strong state involvement in health care, and an assumption that the state should take the lead. In the colonial period private medical practice had not been discouraged, but a network of state services was gradually built up and the dominance of Western medicine was linked to that of the colonial power.

In line with general development ideologies of the period, a belief in the dominant role of the state in health prevailed in the post-Independence era, until undermined in Ghana and Zimbabwe by economic collapse. However, it is important to note that information on utilisation of services, while very scanty, did not support the perception of the state as a lead player in the post-Independence period. If the health system is defined to include the traditional and informal sectors, then it is likely that the majority of ambulatory care in all four countries had always been obtained outside the state sector.

A bias towards hospital and curative care

The colonial heritage in each of the four core countries contributed towards a marked bias towards hospital and curative care, which exists to this day. Government health services in Ghana, dating from the late 1880s, had initially been primarily curative and concerned chiefly with the health of the European population in general and government officials in particular (Dumett 1993; Tsey and Short 1995). In the early part of the twentieth century, colonial health policy became broader in scope, recognising for the first time its responsibility for the health of the indigenous population and the importance of preventive measures in maintaining public health (Patterson 1981). Training of Ghanaian paramedics began in 1917, the number of hospitals gradually increased, a limited number of rural health stations were constructed and infant welfare clinics began to be opened in the 1920s. In the 1940s and 1950s a major hospital building expansion programme got underway. Preventive health services were further strengthened to contain Trypanosomiasis, Yaws and other endemic diseases, but despite this, the pre-Independence health system of the 1950s had a strong emphasis on curative care at fixed centres, the majority of which were in urban areas (Patterson 1981). After Independence in 1957 the curative bias of the health services was accentuated and capacity to deliver preventive services remained very weak (Addae 1997). Although the number of health centres increased quite rapidly post-Independence (Twumasi 1979), access to peripheral health services was still very poor in the late 1970s, and one third of the government health care budget was absorbed by the health services in Greater Accra (IDS Health Group 1978).

The bias towards hospital and curative services was perhaps even stronger in Zimbabwe, since, prior to Independence, separate tertiary hospital services had been established for the white and black populations, resulting in duplication of facilities in the capital. For the white minority, the settler government built comfortable facilities in which care was provided by private doctors, and major hospital facilities in Harare and Bulawayo (Government of the Republic of Zimbabwe 1981). While, from 1979, facilities were no longer segregated officially on racial lines, discrimination based on affordability remained. Preventive services were an early concern of the colonial government, but received a small share of the budget and operated vertically, quite separate from curative services. After Independence the Zimbabwe government tried to correct these biases through increasing access to rural and primary care services, with some considerable success.

Similarly, in Sri Lanka, the colonial government invested in a network of health facilities and public health campaigns (Urageda 1987) but it was not until the post-independence period that the network of primary facilities was considerably expanded through the use of public health midwives and voluntary health workers. In India, the formative 1946 Bhore Committee Report had diagnosed many problems in the health care delivery system of which the bias towards hospital and curative care was one of the most problematic. Since that date many other government reports and policy statements in India have emphasised the importance of shifting resources towards community-based health care. However, while rural public health infrastructure has grown over the decades, the bias towards urban curative care has persisted.

The development of health sector constituencies

With the development of the health sector came the development of various health sector constituencies which shaped and continue to shape health policy. For example, in Ghana, as the government health care system has expanded, so have bureaucratic and professional constituencies which demand more and better facilities, a bigger budget and improved terms and conditions for public sector workers. The general public, despite making extensive use of informal private providers, also represent a powerful pressure to broaden and deepen government health provision. Communities, under 'self-help' initiatives, have contributed to the growth of health infrastructure by constructing health facilities which government was subsequently expected to staff and operate. And politicians in turn have reaped dividends by building or upgrading more and more health facilities, particularly since the reinvigoration of local government in the early 1990s. External donors have bolstered the government's role by channelling the vast majority of their assistance through the public sector. In the Ghanaian context, all the developing constituencies appear to have supported (at least until recently) a central role for the government, and several of the policy groupings have contributed towards the persistent bias towards urban, curative care.

In Sri Lanka the policy groupings interested in health which emerged during the post-war period have rather different origins. They were rooted in the combination of competitive electoral politics, high literacy rates and vocal social movements, and the groupings included emerging trade unions and left-wing political parties. These constituencies also contributed to pressure on the state to adopt responsibility for improving health and social conditions.

Policies on private practice

Chapter 2 described the considerably greater importance of private financing for health care in India and Zimbabwe as compared to the other two core countries. To some extent this difference can be explained by historical analysis of attitudes and policies towards private practice. The fact that Zimbabwe had been a settler colony meant that there had been a market for private medical services during the colonial period, and medical aid societies had developed to finance care for the settler population and workers in the formal sector. The strength of the private sector at Independence had made it very difficult for government to restrict the role of the private sector. More recently low salaries in the government sector and declining quality of public sector services have further boosted private health provision.

In India during the inter-war period a liberal attitude towards private sector growth in health care was adopted: it was common to allow private practice by public doctors and for private doctors to work in public hospitals as 'Honorary Doctors'. By this point in time, a basic regulatory framework for the private sector was in place: the first Medical Registration Acts requiring that all doctors register with the Medical Association were passed between 1912 and 1914. The tendency for many Indians to pay for private medical training for their children, combined with the poor quality of government services, contributed to the continuing importance of the private sector.

Private medical practice in Ghana first developed in the early years of the twentieth century (Tsey and Short 1995), largely practised by expatriate government doctors (Ofosu-Amah 1981, Addae 1997). However, in 1960, the government had banned private practice by government doctors.[2] Those doctors who entered private practice were those whose foreign qualifications were less preferred by government. Hence private practice gained a reputation for low-quality care which it has still not entirely shaken off. Since the 1960s and until recently, the government has largely ignored the existence of the private health sector, concentrating on making publicly funded and provided health services available to all. This attitude was consistent with the general attitude of the government to the private sector (Herbst 1993).

In Sri Lanka rapid growth of the private sector started only about twenty years ago with the initiation of structural adjustment. At this time three factors had contributed to the growth of private practice. First, private practice by government doctors, previously banned, was deregulated in 1976/7. Second, liberalisation of economic policy increased the availability of capital, medical equipment and pharmaceutical imports necessary for private practice. Third, economic growth, coupled with deteriorating quality of government services in terms of waiting times, maintenance, and drug and equipment availability, contributed towards rising demand for private health services.

The state's role in Thailand

Although Thailand has never been colonised, it also has a tradition of strong central government which has its origins in the central authority and administration of the king (Bennett et al. 1998). The Thai national bureaucracy was established by King Rama V in 1892 as part of far reaching reforms aimed at modernising Thai society, and these formed the foundations of the current government system. There had been a degree of government involvement in health care since the nineteenth century, both through public health programmes and training in Western medicine, but until the 1960s there was little explicit government policy relating to health. Since then plans have concentrated on expanding the physical infrastructure, especially in rural areas, and recently on improving resource use and preventive and promotive care. Policy towards the private sector, in line with broader government policies, has been extremely laissez-faire. Private practice by public doctors has always been permitted and widely practised, and the private formal sector was substantial. There has never been a policy of free public care, except for the indigent.

2.2   Economic and social context

Consideration of economic and social factors not only helps to explain trends in health system performance but also provides the broader context in which reform programmes were adopted.

Economic and social indicators

Table 3.1 compares basic economic and social indicators across countries. One of the criteria for country selection was that all core countries should

Table 3.1 Economic and social indicators in the study countries

	Ghana	Zimbabwe	India	Sri Lanka	Thailand
GNP per capita $ (1987 prices)	420	582	454	519	1854
GDP per capita PPP (1987 prices)	1390	1737	1210	1755	5197
% of population below national poverty line*	31.4 (1992)	25.5 (1991)	35.0 (1994)	35.3 (1991)	13.1 (1992)
% of population with <1$ per day**	n/a	41.0	52.5 (1992)	4.0 (1990)	<2%
Government consumption as % GDP	12.34	19.82	10.49	10.44	9.57
Adult illiteracy rate (1995)	35.5	14.9	48.0	9.8	6.2
% population urban	36.4	32.5	27.12	22.4	20.3
Dependency ratio***	0.91	0.83	0.64	0.54	0.47

*   Definition of poverty line is country-specific, based upon local consumption basket and costs.
**   percentage of population living on less than $1 per day at 1985 international prices adjusted for purchasing power parity.
*** Number of dependants/working age population.

Source: World Development Indicators, 1998. 1996 data unless otherwise stated.

be low-income and hence GNP per capita in the core countries was similar, although Zimbabwe had a slightly higher level than the other three. If GDP in terms of purchasing power parity is considered, then Sri Lanka appeared to have a similar income level to Zimbabwe, with Ghana and India having rather lower income levels and Thailand a very much higher level.

An historical representation of GNP growth in the core countries (see Figure 3.1) tells an interesting story. In both Ghana and Zimbabwe, GNP per capita in the early 1970s was considerably higher than in the South Asian countries. However, negative growth in the African countries and positive growth in the South Asian countries (particularly in recent years) has brought about an overall convergence in income levels. Economic decline in Ghana and Zimbabwe has been considerable and one of the key factors leading to deteriorating quality of care in the government sector and stimulating health sector reform.

Poverty rates using the national poverty line were again similar across the core countries, although somewhat lower in Zimbabwe. However,

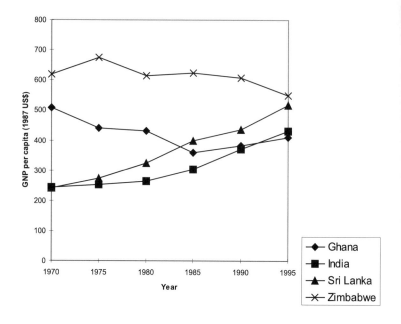

Figure 3.1   Growth in GNP per capita, 1970–95

there were clear differences between countries in terms of the per centage of the population living on less than US $1 per day. Poverty appeared much lower in Sri Lanka than the other core countries, and close to that in Thailand. Unfortunately, data for Ghana were not available. Adult illiteracy rates also varied considerably in the core countries, from a low of 9.8 per cent in Sri Lanka to a high of 48 per cent in India. These differences in social indicators, notably the better social indicators in Sri Lanka, undoubtedly help explain the better health outcomes in Sri Lanka described in the previous chapter.

One potential indicator of the role of government in the economy is the share of GDP spent by government. All four of the core countries had a higher share of GDP being spent by government than Thailand. The role of government in Zimbabwe appeared particularly large, and high levels of taxation in Zimbabwe probably constrained the set of feasible reform options. For example, while social health insurance was frequently discussed in Zimbabwe it was probably not politically viable in the context of existing high tax rates.

Economic and government reform programmes

Figure 3.2 summarises key economic, government and health sector reforms, providing a timeline from 1980. The health sector reforms are discussed in the next section. At the time of the research, all countries had World Bank and IMF-supported economic reform programmes in place, but there were considerable differences in how long these policies had been pursued and the impact they had had upon the health sector.

Ghana's structural adjustment policies were introduced in the early 1980s. While they had had some effect on the health sector (primarily in terms of civil service reform and retrenchment of staff), health reform proposals seem largely to have been internally generated from within the sector. The Ghanaian user-fee policy introduced during the mid-1980s had clearly been driven by financial crisis in the sector, and adopted by the MOH under pressure from the Ministry of Finance (see Chapter 5 for more detail). In Zimbabwe, MOH plans and actions on strengthening cost recovery and introducing contracting out were in conformity with the overall thrust of the Economic and Social Adjustment Programme, which had been introduced in 1991 (civil service reform had started earlier, in 1987).

The Indian government adopted a relatively far-reaching economic reform programme in 1991. The adjustment package had not initially included policies directed at the health sector but none the less it had a significant impact upon the health sector through the tight fiscal environment it generated. The evidence suggested that during the early 1990s the social sectors, particularly health and education, had borne the brunt of the spending cuts associated with the structural adjustment programme. Although central government had managed to maintain its level of health care spending, spending at state level and particularly in the poorer states was considerably below trend in 1991 and 1992 (Jalan and Subbarao 1995). It appeared that cuts had been made to what were supposed to be high-priority programmes: for example, communicable disease control programmes had been subject to greater cuts than medical education (The World Bank 1994).

In Sri Lanka, although economic reform programmes had been in place for many years, the health sector had been little affected and debates on health service reform were only just starting. In Thailand, apart from a very early adjustment and stabilisation programme, the period covered by Figure 3.2 was a period of very considerable economic growth until the

Figure 3.2 Timeline of key economic, government and health reforms, 1980–98

	Ghana	Zimbabwe	India/Tamil Nadu	Sri Lanka	Thailand
1980	-				**Adjustment and stabilisation programme**
1981					Identification cards introduced for fee exemption scheme (LIC)
1982			Publication of First National Health Policy committed government to HFA 2000		
1983	**Economic reform programme introduced**			New Japanese-built hospital given autonomy	
1984					LIC allocation process strengthened
1985	User-fee policy	Health Professions Council established to regulate private sector			
1986					
1987		**Civil service reform**			LIC allocation process strengthened
1988	District strengthening initiative Teaching hospital autonomy bill passed			**Provincial governments established**	
1989					
1990	Implementation of 'cash and carry' for drugs				LIC allocation process strengthened Relaxation of rules for contracting out cleaning Thai Social Security Act introduced contracting fo health care
1991		**Economic and structural adjustment programme**	**Economic reform package**		Tax breaks for hospital investments stopped in BKK Committee to amend Medical Institutions Act established but recommendations not adopted

Year				Divisional level	
1992		User fees revised and enforced more strictly; Government doctors allowed to do private practice	World Bank and GOI began policy dialogue on health; Medical care (for which charges are made) brought under the Consumer Protection Act	strengthed below district; Report of the Presidential Task Force on formulation of a national health policy published	Relaxation of rules for contracting out cleaning
1993			**Constitutional amendment to reinvigorate the Panchayat Raj system of local government**		
1994	MOH HQ restructured	**Cabinet approved contracting out policy**	TN state AIDS control society established		**Cabinet resolution to curtail growth of civil service** Relaxation of rules for contracting out cleaning; MOPH introduced non-private practice allowance for doctors
1995		MOH health reform agenda including restructuring and public private partnerships; Fees withdrawn from health centres; Regulations changed for registration of health institutions	TN medical services corporation established; All medical care brought under Consumer Protection Act		
1996	Ghana health service legislation passed	User-fee retention allowed	TN state blindness control society established; Tamil Nadu tried to introduce visitors' fee in hospitals – later repealed	Brief document entitled 'National Health Policy' published.	
1997	First sector-wide plan and budget implemented	Medical services bill gazetted	Central Council of Health and Family Welfare urged states to strengthen regulation; Law passed on private health care facilities in TN; Bill liberalising insurance market passed	Appointment of Presidential task force on Health Policy Implementation.	**Financial crisis**

	Ghana	Zimbabwe	India/Tamil Nadu	Sri Lanka	Thailand
1998	Piloting of performance contracts within health service and with church hospitals	Contracting out support services programme implemented		Law passed on private medical institutions	Autonomous hospital pilots included in reform package agreed with ADB

Bold type indicates economic and government-wide reforms.

Figure 3.2 (continued)

financial crisis in 1997. Government-wide policies on reducing the size of government were put in place in 1994, but appeared to have relatively little impact on the health sector.

3. Reform policies and plans

All countries, both core countries and Thailand, had been considering reform of their health sectors in recent years, though some had a longer history of reform than others, and some were more advanced in implementation. To a considerable degree, there were common reform themes across all four core countries (and indeed Thailand as well, though from a starting point of a more diversified funding system). The theme were: restructuring the management of public delivery; diversifying funding patterns away from prime dependence on tax revenues to fund public health services; and formalising and increasing relationships between public and private sectors, including revising the framework of rules and regulations relating to the private sector. To at least some degree these themes all drew upon the menu of reforms associated with New Public Management: all implied change in the role of the state and the way that the state carried out its functions in relation to health. These themes are considered in turn next.

3.1 Public sector restructuring

A virtually universal theme was decentralisation, with several of the countries having experienced several waves of decentralisation. Ghana had begun a major effort to strengthen district management in the late 1980s. Planning and management capacities were strengthened, resource management decentralised, and a new cadre of public health doctors trained and appointed to head each district health administration. As they were promoted into regional and ministry posts, there was an important shift of power away from clinical medicine at management and policy levels. In addition, overseas training had exposed key staff to new ideas on health service organisation and financing and this, together with external donor support to management strengthening, helped to explain the 'new public management' language of health sector reform in Ghana. Reform had been extended to the MOH headquarters, and its structure changed to focus on functions rather than professional enclaves. The next step, which had been legislated for, was the creation of a Ghana Health Service which would be managed by an executive agency outside the MOH, enabling the latter to concentrate on its policy-setting and regulatory functions. However, implementation of this reform had been delayed as it conflicted with recent local government legislation which had envisaged all district health services coming under local administrations.

Decentralisation had also been the main thrust of reform proposals in Zimbabwe. Public sector management was generally viewed to be overcentralised, and some decentralisation had already occurred, with a programme of strengthening management and information systems. There were long-term plans to restructure the MOH through decentralisation to a network of purchasers and providers, where purchasers were to be the provincial health offices, and service provision would be managed by a district health management board on behalf of Rural District Councils, and by the hospital boards of provincial and central hospitals.

Sri Lanka had been through two waves of decentralisation. In 1988, a new provincial tier of government had been established with a provincial Health Minister and Department of Health who were responsible for the management of district health services. In 1992, the divisional level below the district had been strengthened. In both cases these changes were government-wide, unlike in Ghana where the initiative came from the Health Ministry. However, despite these changes in formal structure in Sri Lanka, health management remained more centralised than other sectors, in part because the central bureaucracy was very reluctant to relinquish its grip.

In India, the government had enacted an amendment to the constitution in 1993 with the aim of reinvigorating the *Pachayat raj* system of local government. This system operated councils at district, block and village levels which should ultimately adopt responsibility for a variety of local level functions, including health care. However, few had as yet taken over this responsibility, due to resistance from higher levels of the system.

These four countries provided an interesting contrast. In three (India, Sri Lanka and Zimbabwe to a more limited extent) reforms to the health sector were part of broader government reforms to strengthen provincial and local government. Indeed, in Sri Lanka, the MOH was a reluctant follower. In Ghana, in contrast, the changes were driven by the MOH, and indeed ran counter to longer-term government plans to place the management of district health services within local government structures. Perhaps because of MOH leadership, reforms had proceeded faster in Ghana than elsewhere, notably India, where there had been very limited implementation (except in four states with a World Bank-supported programme of reform). In Zimbabwe there had been very limited implementation of the broader structural reforms (though more progress with specific reforms internal to the health sector discussed below).

In terms of the specific model of decentralisation, Zimbabwe, the Government of Ghana and India proposed reforms involving devolution to a local government system, whereas the Ghana MOH and Sri Lanka were pursuing deconcentration of the MOH to lower administrative levels. As with the core countries, Thailand was seeking to strengthen lower management levels within the public health system hierarchy. As in Sri Lanka, the model was one of deconcentration rather than devolution, and the highly centralised political system had not encouraged the development of strong and independent lower systems of government.

3.2   Diversifying funding

The two African countries had sought to diversify funding for the public sector health services by imposing or increasing user fees. In both countries this was a response to economic crisis. Both countries had also been actively considering the introduction of compulsory social insurance for the formal sector. In contrast, despite shortages of tax funds for public health services, neither India nor Sri Lanka had adopted a user fee policy nor actively explored other sources of funds such as the introduction or expansion of compulsory insurance. Thailand, like other middle income countries in its region, had implemented a compulsory social insurance programme for private sector workers. It had also progressively refined its scheme for exempting the poor from the fees charged in public facilities. Chapter 5 further explores user fee reform and explanations for differences between countries.

3.3   Relationships between public and private sectors

While reshaping relationships between public and private sectors was under discussion in all the countries, plans were at a much earlier stage than with either of the other two themes. In no country had there been consideration of fundamentally transforming the scope of government involvement in the health sector, nor of significantly changing the public/private mix. Although there had been important changes in the balance of public and private services in recent decades in all the countries, this had been the result of unplanned, rather than planned change. In all four core countries, public opinion and the views of public sector workers seemed to be significant constraints on government action to alter purposefully the balance between public and private providers. This did not seem to be the case in Thailand, where the overall climate of opinion, both within government and in the country at large, was much more sympathetic to the private sector. India was a partial exception, in that there was significant mistrust of the public sector amongst the public at large, though public health workers were a powerful force in favour of the status quo.

As discussed in Chapter 7, strengthening the regulatory powers of the government (and states in India) was a theme in all countries, though with only some limited progress. In Ghana, Sri Lanka and Thailand, revisions to the regulatory framework for health services were still under discussion; in Zimbabwe some changes had already been made and others were proceeding through Parliament, and in Tamil Nadu a new law had been passed but was encountering implementation difficulties. In all countries, vested interests were a powerful constraint on change, especially where public sector staff – often at all levels, from the Minister downwards – benefited from the lack of control of private medical facilities.

4.   Reform processes

4.1   Forces for and against change

Government actors outside the Ministry of Health were commonly identified as the initiators of change, partly because the declining macro-economic situation affected the state more generally. In Zimbabwe, for example, reforms such as contracting out had been put on the policy agenda by the Public Service Commission as part of a drive to reduce the size of the civil service. Similarly in Thailand, contracting out had also been driven by actors external to the MOH, particularly the civil service commission, aiming to stop the growth of public sector employment. In Ghana, the Ministry of Finance had proved to be an ally to the MOH in supporting an increase in user fees, as it saw that this would increase government revenue collections.

In terms of the supporters or proponents of reform, in virtually all countries (perhaps with the partial exception of Sri Lanka) there appeared to be an alliance between technocrats within the Ministry of Health and the technical advisors of donor and international organisations. The relative roles of these two sets of actors varied between countries.

In India, the leaders of reform programmes at the state level appeared to be senior civil servants frustrated by apathy within the bureaucracy. In some states, international players such as the World Bank and DFID were engaged in supporting state-level reform programmes. It was in these states that reforms had been most marked and rapid. In other states such as Tamil Nadu, without such externally supported reform programmes, the role of external actors had been quite limited.

In Ghana, actors within the MOH were seen as the prime players: technocrats at both the central and regional level had played a key part in pushing the reform programme, but here too international organisations had played an important role in financing and endorsing reforms. In Zimbabwe, policy-makers within the MOH on the whole endorsed the recommendations and used the same discourse as the international actors. However, it was unclear how committed they were to actual implementation of the reforms.

In Thailand, there had been far less of a comprehensive reform agenda articulated and no clear ideological stance to reforms. However techno-crats within the MOPH had played an important role in shaping the reforms. International agencies were much less important in this context, though the ADB had recently gained leverage through its support during the financial crisis.

Health workers were a powerful group of actors whose position varied considerably by policy and by country. In India, health workers were important opponents of many reforms: government health workers had opposed contracting out (for fear of job losses), user fees (for fear of loss of informal user charge revenue) and regulation (for fear of tighter controls upon private sector practice by government workers). In Zimbabwe, the broader programme of economic reform had had adverse effects for many government employees and had resulted in a series of strikes within the health sector (1988, 1989, 1994 and twice during 1996) (Mutizwa-Mangiza 1997). Probably partly because of this conflict and the perceived connection between the structural adjustment programme and health sector reforms, the latter had also encountered opposition from health workers. In Ghana, health workers appeared more inclined to support reforms: they certainly had seen increases in user fees as a way to increase revenues and hence service quality, and regional staff had supported decentralisation.

Particular elements of the reform agenda had generated support or opposition from specific groups of actors affected by the policy. For example, private sector practitioners and their representative bodies had contributed significantly to the shaping and success (or failure) of regulatory policies. Similarly central level bureaucrats had been important players with regard to decentralisation policies. Each of the following four chapters considers in more detail the perspective of different interest groups with respect to the four tracer policies.

4.2 Phasing and implementing reforms

In Ghana, it was notable that reforms had been introduced incrementally, without a comprehensive agenda of reform (Cassells and Janovsky 1996). A key explanation is likely to be that they had not been championed politically, requiring civil servants to proceed opportunistically. Even a strategic planning exercise in 1997 had not sought to build consensus around a clear set of policy proposals, but rather almost regarded consultation and consensus as an end in itself. It is perhaps not surprising, therefore, that reforms in Ghana had been mainly concerned with improving the management and functioning of government health services rather than transforming the scope of government involvement in the health sector or significantly changing the public/private mix.

In contrast, the reforms in Zimbabwe were more radical, embodying a more comprehensive and innovative restructuring of relationships within the public sector and with the private sector; however, it was unclear to what extent the grand restructuring plan would actually be implemented, and the proposals seemed to be internally generated to a lesser extent than was the case with Ghana.

In India, achieving change was particularly complex because of the multiple levels of government: change could not simply be dictated from the centre and state governments had substantial discretion with regard to health. The reform process had tended to be one of coalition-building or focused on demonstration projects, and the pace of reform had differed substantially between the states. However, in some states such as Tamil Nadu, some NPM-type reforms were being introduced quite rapidly. The key constraint on the pace of change in India appeared to be less the capacity to plan and manage reforms, and more a few key obstacles and especially the threat of opposition from organised labour.

Thailand presented quite a contrast. There was a strong, professionally-driven commitment to expanding basic services through the public sector to the low-income population but also a notable openness to the private heath market and involvement of public sector employees in that market. NPM tools were used in a selective manner: to contract out for non-clinical services (but not to attempt system-wide reform using a contracting model); and to allow a certain degree of independence to hospitals whilst stopping short of full-scale autonomy. An incremental and centralised approach to reform may have been at least partly due to an organisational culture characterised by high power distances, lack of value given to innovation and lack of strong political leadership. It remained to be seen whether the 1997 financial crisis would stimulate more radical thinking and change.

Reform paths had also been affected by political in/stability. In Zimbabwe (perhaps partly because of the lack of internal ownership of reforms) there had been problems of inconsistent policy direction. For example, the Cabinet had abandoned its policy on contracting out just prior to elections – although this policy had later (post-elections) been reintroduced. In Thailand there had been very frequent political change, but the bureaucracy seemed remarkably buffered from the effects of change, and political upheaval generally did not result in anything other than minor changes in health policy. However, this lack of political control of policy may have been a contributing factor to the lack of an overall reform agenda.

In none of the case study countries had reforms been politically driven or associated with political transformation. Hence the circumstances in case study countries differed considerably from countries such as Zambia, South Africa and Colombia where reform programmes have been more all-encompassing and supported by strong political commitment (CHP and HEU 1999, Yepes and Sanchez in press).

5. The relevance of alternative theories

The key features of the health systems which had evolved in the five countries studied included:

- a strong state role in both the financing and provision of health care;
- a strong parallel and separate private health sector;
- limited crossover between public and private sectors: for example, weak regulation, and limited government purchasing of care from private providers.

Health sector reform in the study countries emphasised decentralisation, the diversification of funding and restructuring of public and private relationships. How relevant are the theoretical frameworks described in Chapter 1 to explaining both the status quo and the reforms in the study countries?

5.1 Neoclassical economics

Neoclassical economics offers a number of rationales for state intervention in the health sector, including the presence of externalities and public goods, asymmetric information, insurance market imperfections and problems of market structure (see Annex to Chapter 1). None of these appeared to offer satisfactory explanations for the pattern of state intervention observed.

The theory of externalities and public goods suggests that the epidemiological profile of a country will affect appropriate government roles. All four core countries exhibited a pattern of disease where infectious and parasitic disease dominated, while Thailand had the disease profile of a middle-income country, with heart disease, accidents and cancers accounting for the top three causes of death and rising sharply since the late 1980s (Ministry of Public Health, Thailand 1997). In the core countries this epidemiological pattern may justify a strong state role, but the necessary state role to offset such a market failure primarily encompasses primary care, and preventive and promotive health activities. In practice the state's role was far broader than that, and indeed notably biased in favour of curative care delivered through hospitals.

Problems associated with asymmetric information, particularly between patient and health care provider, were widespread. It seems plausible that low literacy rates are associated with higher degrees of market failure. In Ghana nearly half the adult population had never been to school and less than half of adults were literate (GSS 1995). Literacy rates were lower still in India. Consumer information was therefore limited, especially as regards Western health care. In the absence of internal or external mechanisms to assure quality of care and professional ethics, providers were unlikely to be good agents for patients. Even in the other study countries where literacy rates were higher, policy makers still considered lack of information amongst consumers to be a problem. However, it was not viewed as a reason for sole state provision.

Considerable imperfections in the market for health insurance were apparent. For example, in Ghana commercial health insurance barely existed: there was only one company which offered medical insurance and the benefit package was quite limited. In Zimbabwe, unusually for Sub-Saharan Africa, there was a substantial insurance sector based on not-for-profit insurance which had seen rapid growth since independence. However, it covered only the middle- and higher-income workers, neglecting even the lower-income workers in the formal sector. In India, health insurance was largely limited to the formal sector (Ellis, Alam and Gupta 1996) with compulsory schemes for government workers and poor factory workers. The General Insurance Company had a monopoly on private insurance (though the industry is being deregulated), and only a further 1.8 million were covered by its medical insurance policies. There were some innovative insurance schemes in rural areas offered by NGOs, but total population coverage was very low. The situation was broadly similar in Sri Lanka, though private health insurance firms were allowed to operate. In Thailand, the private insurance market was extremely small, even before the advent of the compulsory social insurance scheme.

Thus in no country did private insurance offer reasonable protection against risk and uncertainty even for better-off groups, while affordability would put it out of reach of the bulk of the population. These widespread limitations of private insurance create the rationale for public intervention to finance health care. Public financing need not mean public provision, yet in the study countries, with the partial exception of Thailand, integrated public financing and provision was the dominant mode of service delivery.

Market structure arguments do not constitute a powerful justification of state involvement in provision, except at early stages of hospital development. In low-income countries and areas, the private sector largely supplies outpatient care from units of small size – usually a single provider – and consumers have considerable choice as in India or Ghana. However the underdevelopment of capital markets and limited access to capital can be a potential barrier to entry in the hospital sector. Moreover hospitals often have local monopolies, which can create concern if they seek to exploit this position (as was suggested for a mine hospital contracted to provide care for the local population in Zimbabwe: McPake and Hongoro 1995). Where the private market is quite fully developed, as in Thailand, there does appear to be substantial competition between hospitals and considerable consumer choice in large urban centres (Bennett 1997a, Muraleedharan 1999).

Thus neoclassical economics had little power to explain current patterns of financing and provision. This does not negate its potential relevance as a normative guide; however, it is significant that countries did not appear to acknowledge its relevance in their decisions on desired patterns. While reform agendas emphasised restructuring public/private relationships, decisions rarely seemed to be driven by arguments derived from neoclassical economics. The institutional analysis associated with New Institutional Economics appeared to offer far better explanations for reform strategies and progress.

5.2 New institutional economics

The historical analysis presented earlier suggests that the notion of 'path dependence', with institutional change occurring only slowly and incrementally, does offer insights into the existing role of the state in study countries. During the colonial period there had been substantial investment in curative facilities. This helped determine standards and expectations in the newly independent countries. Consequently developments during the post-Independence period emphasised the further expansion and development of a curative care network. Similarly in some countries, such as Zimbabwe, liberal policies towards the private sector during the colonial period made it difficult to enforce any tighter regulations at a later date.

North's theory of institutions considers not only the explicit rules which make up institutions but also the implicit or informal rules: 'the codes of conduct, norms of behaviour and conventions' (North 1990: 36). The studies found that there were frequently strong informal rules in the study countries concerning equity of access to health care. These appeared quite powerful in terms of explaining current patterns of state intervention. In Ghana, for example, most people would assert that a woman is entitled to the care necessary to prevent death in childbirth, whether or not she can afford it (Smithson, Asamoa-Baah and Mills 1997). The same applies to a child who requires life-saving treatment. Individual cases of life-threatening illness commonly received high-profile media coverage and attracted donations from the public to cover the cost of care. Thus it was widely felt by the general population that health care should not be available solely for those willing and able to pay.

In Sri Lanka the constitution required that every citizen had access to adequate health care and there was a strong commitment to equity:

> The commitment to provide comprehensive promotive, preventive, curative and rehabilitative health care, free of direct cost and within easy access to the entire population, has been the fundamental premise on which successive governments based actions for meeting the health needs of the people. (Russell and Attanayake 1997: 4)

Equity arguments were incorporated into the discourse of the trade union movement very early on, and this and public pressure for public service provision remained important.

Public commitment to equity appeared somewhat weaker in India. While health care was seen in official policy statements as a basic right, and the government role to be fundamental in securing this right for the whole population, there was an enormous gap between intent and practice. Consequently, people did not trust the government to provide good quality curative care, as demonstrated by the views from a focus group discussion:

> Honestly, we have no hope. We have tried it over the past years. We even tried bringing pressure through political parties. There is something basic that is wrong. This has lead us to decide – private is best. Not as a choice but due to necessity. (Rakodi 1998)

Other branches of New Institutional Economics also offer insights into explanations for the dominant state role in provision. Reasons probably lay both with the entrenched power of groups involved with public provision, and the difficulties of arranging and controlling provision by private providers. As discussed at more length in Chapter 6, the transactions costs associated with purchasing private sector care can be considerable and are increased when there is a lack of trust between parties (as there commonly was between public and private sectors) and when the product being purchased is complex (as health care certainly is) and hence quality is difficult to monitor. Faced with high transaction costs, lack of trust and fear of quality-reducing opportunist behaviour by the private sector, combining both the financing and production of services within the public sector may be a rational decision.

Approaches in Thailand to offsetting some of the key problems of asymmetric information placed emphasis on worker education, but also considered a range of broader approaches to ensuring ethical and accountable behaviour including monitoring by the social security office, encouraging quality assurance within the medical professions and hospital industry, introducing a scheme for accreditation of hospitals, and encouraging an active and informed media (Mills et al. 1999). These mechanisms for encouraging broader accountability on the part of health care providers seem to draw more from the discussions of exit, voice and hierarchy in new institutional economics than the arguments of neo-liberal economics.

5.3 Theories of bureaucracy and public choice

In all five countries examined, the traditional structure of the Ministry of Health drew considerably upon Weberian ideas regarding bureaucracy: Ministries of Health tended to be hierarchical, with substantial bodies of rules and regulations governing operations at different levels within the hierarchy. However the Ministries examined clearly fell well short of Weber's ideal bureaucracy: to differing degrees they suffered from resource shortages, lack of expertise and lack of clarity about rules and regulations. Certainly, differences in these aspects between countries contributed to differences in performance in the health sector. The general trend towards decentralisation in the study countries suggests that there was an increasing sense that decision-making within the health sector was too hierarchical (and possibly too rule-bound) and that this was impeding effective service delivery.

There also appeared to be differences between countries in the extent to which the private preferences of government employees influenced their behaviour within the work context. For example, as discussed in the previous chapter, quite substantial differences between countries were observed in the extent to which public sector doctors adhered to regulations governing private practice. In India, for example, some public sector workers pursued their own interests and paid little heed to public sector rules, and in general this was detrimental to public sector performance. Thus public choice theory appears of relevance in that context, though its broader relevance to all countries was questionable.

6. Conclusions

The influence of colonial administrations helped establish state domination of the formal health sector early in the core countries. Of the four, only in Zimbabwe was there much presence of private Western medical practitioners during the colonial regime, a result of the settlers market. Although the colonial administrations created public health structures to cope with infectious disease and epidemics, they were under-resourced compared to curative care, and hence set the pattern of curative care domination and especially hospitals. A basic network of facilities was extended to the rural population (except in Zimbabwe where this was left to the missions to do, outside settler areas), but the primacy of the need to serve the colonial administration biased allocation of resources.

Newly independent states sought to address the legacies of inequalities, and in so doing accentuated the curative bias of the inherited health systems (with the exception of the more recently independent Zimbabwe). In accordance with the dominant ideology of the time, they also accentuated state domination in the health sector, in the process creating and strengthening groups which had vested interests in maintaining the state's position. Similarly, they gave little attention to the private sector.

In the two African countries, economic crisis, the expansion of state services beyond the ability of the country to maintain and supply them, and the persuadings of external agencies, had forced a reconsideration of the role of the state in recent years. However, in general reforms were nibbling away at the fringes of the state, rather than fundamentally changing its role in health. This was even more true in India and Sri Lanka: in Sri Lanka the public sector was still firmly entrenched as the preferred mode of service provision, and few reforms had been introduced, other than some limited degree of decentralisation; in India, the public sector seemed to have widely lost the trust of the general population, but had great difficulty reinventing itself.

These political economy explanations for the observed dominance of the state in formal health policy appear convincing in explaining the state's role and reasons for intervention. However, it should not be forgotten that while documentation and policies focused on the formal health system, use of other providers was widespread, yet largely ignored until very recently. From the perspective of the population at large, public providers were only one of their options, and usually not the preferred one if they had money to pay for private care.

In terms of the relevance of the alternative theories in explaining the role of government in the study countries, the most important influence appeared to be the institutional configurations which different countries had inherited (path dependence). Historical factors are important as they help determine both the technically feasible set of reform options (based upon existing organisational structures) and the politically feasible set of reform options (based upon existing interest groups and informal norms). None the less all of the frameworks outlined in Chapter 1 had some relevance to understanding the existing situation and reform options.

4
Bureaucratic Commercialisation: Decentralisation of Hospital Management

1. Introduction

An emphasis on decentralisation characterises most components of the international health sector reform agenda, from user fees and contracting out to more radical proposals for a purchaser/provider split. One of the most common reforms advocated by donors to improve management performance and efficiency is the decentralisation of Ministry of Health structures, usually to the district level, but also to large hospitals through the establishment of hospital management boards which have considerable management autonomy (McPake 1996; World Bank 1993). The latter reform, which can be seen as the introduction of more commercial styles of management into public bureaucracies and is often termed 'hospital autonomy', is the subject of this chapter.

The next section briefly reviews the economic and institutional arguments for greater hospital autonomy that are grounded in the new public management agenda, and the basic concept of autonomy in general. Section 3 looks at the nature and extent of this policy across the case study countries, policy rationales and the degree to which autonomy was implemented in practice. Section 4 then briefly asks whether greater management autonomy led to improved service performance, since performance can shed light on the organisation's capacity to provide services. However, it should be noted that this was only a minor part of the research because policy was largely undeveloped in practice. The main focus of the research was on MOH capacity to develop and implement policy, which is examined in section 5. Given the limited extent of hospital autonomy across the five countries, the most relevant question concerned capacity constraints which might explain why hospital autonomy had not reached the policy agenda, or why implementation had been delayed. The chapter ends by drawing conclusions on the process of policy development and capacity strengthening.

2. Hospital autonomy: why and what?

Ideas for hospital autonomy in developing countries have been informed by health sector reform in industrialised countries, notably the UK, and influenced by bilateral and multilateral donors (McPake 1996). The rationales which underlie the reform are economic and institutional and form part of the new public management reform agenda, founded on the assumption that a centralised bureaucracy makes hospital management inefficient, inflexible and unresponsive to users (Bennett, Russell and Mills 1996). Proponents of greater hospital autonomy argue it will achieve the following:

1. *Address inefficiency.* Large hospitals, often tertiary hospitals, have been targeted for reform because they consume a high proportion of the national health budget and are often the most inefficient parts of the health system (Barnum and Kutzin 1993; World Bank 1993). If tertiary hospital administrators are not responsible for financial decisions or their consequences, they have no incentive to identify wasteful practices, no authority to address and use resources more efficiently. The proposed solution is to delegate greater financial responsibility to hospital managers and make them more accountable for their resource decisions, thereby generating incentives to use resources more efficiently.
2. *Increase flexibility and innovation.* The existing centralised and bureaucratic organisational environment within Ministries of Health is argued to be restrictive and stifling, preventing flexible resource use and adoption of new management systems and practices. The proposed solution is to extract hospital management from this environment to stimulate innovation. Being able to appoint experienced private sector managers to hospital management boards to improve management practices is also seen as a potential benefit of the policy.
3. *Make management more responsive.* A common critique of central bureaucracies is that they are unresponsive and unaccountable service providers which do not respond to people's needs (Mackintosh 1992). Decentralised management may address this problem because managers will be closer to service delivery and patients, particularly if community or user 'voice' is represented on the management board.
4. *Shift the burden of operational management away from the centre.* This would release central staff to focus on policy and strategic management roles.

These arguments were of relevance to the case study countries, albeit to differing degrees, since in all of them the MOH organisation was a centralised bureaucracy which placed strict limits on hospital managers' financial responsibilities and flexibility, contributing to service performance weaknesses within the bureaucracy.

A policy to decentralise management authority to hospital boards raises difficult organisational and political questions and demands new management capacities at the central MOH and at hospital level. The nature of the implementation problems to a large extent depend on (a) the degree of decision-making authority which the policy aims to decentralise, and (b) the type and range of management functions to be decentralised.

In the literature, different forms of decentralisation are commonly referred to as deconcentration, devolution, delegation and privatisation (Table 4.1). While each form can be implemented to a greater or lesser degree, the four categories represent a spectrum of decentralised decision-making power. Policies on hospital management relate most closely to the delegation form of decentralisation, where management authority is given to an organisation not directly controlled by the central government ministry. In principle, this involves handing over a relatively high degree of decision-making authority.

Two broad types of delegation can be distinguished. Delegation to autonomous bodies, or autonomisation, involves the transfer of key management decision-making powers to a board of management, including the ability to raise and retain some revenue. However, the hospital remains subject to hierarchical supervision, is funded to a considerable degree by government subsidies, and operates on a non-profit basis with limited commercial objectives. Delegation to corporate bodies, or corporatisation, is a more radical strategy where managers have virtually complete control over all aspects, and the hospital's survival is dependent on its ability to raise revenue. The hospital remains in public ownership, but provision of care to 'public' patients may be specifically purchased by the state rather than ensured through a general budget subsidy.

Since both autonomisation and corporatisation affect a number of dimensions of hospital functioning, each of which may be decentralised to different degrees, there is in practice no clear distinction between the various organisational forms, with the traditional centralised management approach shading into autonomisation as hospitals are given greater authority, into corporatisation, and finally into privatisation (Harding and Preker 1999).

Table 4.1 A spectrum of autonomy

Deconcentration	Devolution	Delegation to autonomous / corporate bodies	Privatisation
← least -------------------------------------- spectrum of decentralisation --------------------------------- most →			
Some administrative functions moved 'down' the line Ministry to sub-national Ministry offices.	Creation of sub-national government and administrative structures with sub-national government departments.	Transfer of management responsibility for defined functions to a public organisation located outside the central line ministry.	Sale of government assets and transfer of management responsibility to newly created or existing private organisations, with no direct government control.

Source: adapted from Mills et al. (1990).

3.   Policy and practice

3.1   Policy

Decentralisation of hospital management was more firmly on the policy agenda in Ghana and Zimbabwe than in India or Sri Lanka (see Table 4.2). Policy development was most advanced in Ghana and it was the only case study country with legislation that made Hospital Boards legal, corporate entities. The first piece of legislation was the 1988 Hospital Administration Law (PNDC Law 209), which established Teaching Hospital Boards at the two main teaching hospitals, Korle Bu (KBTH) in Accra and Komfo Anokye (KATH) in Kumasi. On paper the Boards were 'bodies corporate' with the 'power to sue and be sued in their corporate name' and 'acquire, hold and dispose of property and to enter into any other contract or transaction'. They were granted extensive management powers, including the right to 'appoint staff and determine remuneration and benefits of such staff' and to 'recommend to the Secretary [Minister] the scale of fees to be paid by patients'. Progress with policy implementation was, however, negligible until 1995, but since then there has been some management decentralisation to the Boards (see below). A second piece of legislation passed in 1996, the Ghana Health Service and Teaching Hospitals Act (Act 525), strengthened the legal status of the Boards and clarified their organisational structure and functions.

In Zimbabwe hospital autonomy was only at proposal stage and management of the four main tertiary hospitals in Harare and Bulawayo remained centralised. These hospitals once enjoyed a greater degree of autonomy under the Salisbury Hospitals Act (1975) but, after Independence, the Act was amended in 1981 to return hospital management to the control of the central MOHCW. More recently discussions on health sector reform, heavily influenced by donor advocacy and advice, revived hospital autonomy as an integral component of wider reform proposals that involved a total restructuring of the centralised system through a purchaser/provider split (MOHCW 1996). In the proposals, central and provincial MOHCW offices would act as purchasers, responsible for defining needs, setting priorities and, through contractual arrangements with providers, allocating resources and monitoring performance. Above the district level, provincial and central hospitals with Hospital Boards of Management would act as providers and be delegated autonomy or 'trust' status.

In the South Asian case study countries, hospital autonomy was not on the policy agenda, with tertiary hospital management highly centralised and no prospect for change in the near future. But the research identified

Table 4.2 The extent of national hospital autonomy policy, and organisations considered by the research

Country	National policy on hospital autonomy	Organisations considered	Legislation
Ghana	Yes	The two government teaching hospitals: • Korle Bu in Accra • Komfo Anokye in Kumasi	Hospital Administration Law (PNDC Law 209), 1988 Ghana Health Service and Teaching Hospitals Act, 1996
Zimbabwe	No: proposed		
India	No	• Tamil Nadu Medical Supply Corporation	1995 Companies Act
		• Tamil Nadu State AIDS Control Society	Tamil Nadu Societies Registration Act
		• Tamil Nadu State Blindness Control Society	1986 Act of State Government
		• Andhra Pradesh Council for Hospital Management	
Sri Lanka	No	• Sri Jayawardenapura General Hospital	Sri Jayawardena General Hospital Act No. 54, 1983
Thailand	No	• All hospitals	

several autonomous organisations in India and Sri Lanka which had the potential to provide insights into organisational autonomy and related government capacity questions.

In Tamil Nadu (TN) three autonomous organisations were identified: TN Medical Supply Corporation (TNMSC); TN State Aids Control Society (TNSACS), and TN State Blindness Control Society (TNBCS). The former was a government-owned corporation established in 1995 under the Companies Act and the other two were non-profit organisations established in the mid-1990s under the Tamil Nadu Societies Registration Act. In addition, an evaluation of the relatively autonomous Andhra Pradesh Council for Hospital Management (Andhra Pradesh Vaidya Vidhan Parishad, or APVVP) by Chawla and George (1996) is drawn upon here where relevant performance and capacity questions arise. APVVP was established by a 1986 Act of the Andhra Pradesh state government and was a parastatal organisation responsible for the management of 162 district and other secondary hospitals. It replaced the branch of the Department of Health previously responsible for hospital administration.

In Sri Lanka one exceptional case of relative hospital autonomy was identified at Sri Jayarwardenapura General Hospital (SJGH). This was a government teaching hospital, built and equipped in the early 1980s with Japanese capital grants, and given corporate status by the Sri Jayarwardenapura General Hospital Act No. 54 of 1983. This hospital was an anomaly in the system, in particular because it was the only government facility in the country which could set and retain user fees.

In Thailand hospital autonomy was not under discussion at the time of the research, possibly due to the relative financial autonomy already enjoyed by hospitals which stemmed from their control over substantial user fee revenue. However, the 1997 economic crisis and resulting greater donor leverage stimulated more debate on the desirability of increased hospital management autonomy. This accorded with trends elsewhere in the public sector: a new public service reform bill on 'Executing Agencies' had been drafted which would allow ministries to create new forms of public organisation, located outside or some distance from bureaucratic structures and regulations. Public hospitals were one of the possibilities for more autonomous management and establishing a pilot autonomous hospital was a condition of an ADB Social Sector Policy Loan.

3.2   Rationales and objectives

Two main types of rationale appear to have driven policy. First, there was a desire for greater freedom to mobilise resources through user fees or other commercial projects in order to maintain basic service standards following budget cutbacks, or to promote centres of 'medical excellence'. Funding shortages in Ghana and the medical elite's aspirations to maintain service standards had created the need 'to formulate policies and develop plans and strategies to make the Teaching Hospitals self-financing' (Law 209). APVVP was also a response to a funding crisis and the need to improve poor standards in rural hospitals through an autonomous body with more freedom to generate revenue through commercial projects and user fees (Chawla and George 1996). The state government may also have wanted to use APVVP to distance itself from poorly performing hospitals and an impending decision to introduce user fees. In Sri Lanka autonomy was granted to SJGH so that fees could be charged to help finance 'a centre of national and international medical excellence' with higher operational costs.

A second and more recent rationale underlying autonomy proposals appears to be more closely linked to the NPM agenda. As well as autonomy to raise revenue, emphasis was placed on the need to generate better management and greater efficiency by making hospital managers responsible for their resource decisions, and, in the case of the proposed purchaser/provider split in Zimbabwe, more accountable through the contracts and performance monitoring which autonomy would entail.

In Ghana, policy changes had been driven since 1995 by a perceived need to strengthen management decision-making. In 1995 and 1996 the two teaching hospitals were granted greater control over non-staff recurrent spending following approval from the Ministry of Finance and the Controller and Accountant General to operate on a subvented (block grant) basis (Smithson, Asamoa-Baah and Mills 1997). Any savings from this grant could be retained rather than returned to the Treasury (Larbi 1998).

Policy-makers in both countries were operating within a macro-policy context of structural adjustment and associated proposals and pressure for reform of government organisations through autonomisation, corporatisation or privatisation. While the specific emphasis on hospital autonomy can be associated with the spread of reform ideas from industrialised countries, notably the UK, and donor pressure, in Ghana the MOH also played a proactive role, for example, pursuing a policy of deconcentration in general, restructuring the budget to transfer control of resources to sub-national cost centres, and strengthening regional and district management levels. In this context greater financial autonomy for the teaching hospitals was a logical part of the decentralisation process (Smithson, Asamoa-Baah and Mills 1997).

The NPM agenda also appeared to have influenced reform in Tamil Nadu. The AIDS and Blindness Control Societies, funded by the World Bank through central government, were granted autonomy on the grounds that they needed greater financial and management flexibility to be able to work closely and effectively with NGOs (Bennett and Muraleedharan 1998). In the case of the TN Medical Supply Corporation, autonomy was simply a strategy to improve radically the dire management of pharmaceutical supply for government hospitals.

3.3   Organisational arrangements and accountability

The official organisational arrangements for autonomy set out under the legislation in Ghana, India and Sri Lanka had several similarities. For each organisation, a board or governing body responsible for overall management was established, accountable to the Minister of Health through the Secretary of Health. One common feature of these boards was their composition, which largely consisted of senior government officials from central ministries. In India, the TNMSC was chaired by the Secretary of Health and composed of senior MOH officials. Similarly the President of both the TN AIDS and Blindness Control Societies was the Secretary of Health, and their governing bodies included senior officials from different government departments. The hospital boards in Ghana and Sri Lanka were also composed of senior MOH officials, although medical professionals from the hospital also sat on the boards.

Across the countries, with the exception of Ghana, there was no place on the boards for people with private sector management experience or representatives of users and the wider community. Board composition in itself, dominated as it was by senior bureaucrats, was therefore likely to limit the impact of greater autonomy. In Ghana, both boards included prominent businessmen with extensive private sector experience.

Across countries, the Minister had the power to appoint the chairperson of the board and most of its members. Under the 1996 Act in Ghana, all members of the board were appointed by the President. In Sri Lanka the Chairman and five other board members were appointed by the Minister, including the Hospital Director responsible for day-to-day management of the hospital. Similarly in the Indian organisations, the chairman and governing body were appointed by the Minister.

Legislation in each country gave the Minister a great deal of control, and not only over board composition. Boards' functions and powers were subject to ministerial directives. Thus in Ghana the legislation in 1988 and 1996 stated that the 'functions of a Teaching Hospital Board under this Act shall be exercised subject to such policy directives as the Minister may determine', and user-fee levels could notably only be set by the Board 'subject to the approval of the Minister'. Similar clauses existed in the 1983 Act for SJGH and the APVVP legislation.

In principle, therefore, organisational arrangements left substantial control in the hands of the Minister and room for both political and bureaucratic interference in day-to-day management. Consequently, the degree of autonomy was likely to depend on the political norms and practices in each country; in a culture of political interference autonomy might be extremely limited in practice.

3.4   Autonomy in practice

The autonomy granted to teaching hospitals in Ghana, to APVVP in India and to SJGH in Sri Lanka was indeed, in practice, more limited than that set out in policy frameworks. For example, in Ghana, the 1988 Hospital Boards were not inaugurated until 1990 and the policy remained largely unimplemented until 1995:

> Beyond the formal change in governance of the hospital there remained little qualitative difference between the management of KATH [and KBTH] in 1995 and what prevailed in 1988. [T]he Board, the hospital management and the Ministry of Health all consider that the hospital does not, at present, enjoy any significant degree of autonomy. (Smithson, Asamoa-Baah and Mills 1997: 36)

At APVVP, although the creation of an arm's length agency had structural advantages for the Department of Health (it only needed to deal with one umbrella organisation rather than over 160 hospitals) the arrangement did not alter management roles or incentives at hospital level since hospital managers' decision-making powers were not increased. And in Sri Lanka, while SJGH enjoyed more autonomy than other hospitals due to its block grant and user-fee revenue, the hospital's management was heavily constrained by political considerations and interference.

The degree of autonomy that hospital managers actually enjoyed in the five case study countries is summarised below for the main management functions.

Strategic management

In general, the autonomous organisations studied lacked responsibility for defining their overall mission, broad strategic goals and objectives. Only the exceptional autonomous organisations in Sri Lanka and India had developed a mission statement of their own, set organisational aims and objectives, or adopted new management systems and relationships with the private sector.

Human resource management

In all four core countries and in Thailand, hospital managers had little latitude over human resource management. Core staff establishment levels in hospitals were centrally set by the Ministry of Finance and Public Service Commission in each country, and the Public Service Commission also controlled recruitment, remuneration, promotion, transfer and discipline of all medical staff.

Although centralised human resource management was a common barrier to greater autonomy, there was more room for manoeuvre in Thailand and at SJGH in Sri Lanka due to user-fee revenue. In Thailand, fee revenue made up about 50 per cent of hospital recurrent expenditure and gave managers flexibility to recruit extra staff on a temporary basis, including doctors. Similarly at SJGH, fee revenue made up 30 per cent of recurrent expenditure and could be used to recruit ancillary staff and pay higher salaries to medical staff. The Board could also select and appoint medical staff rapidly through its own advertisements if there was a vacancy for an already established position, but had to seek Treasury approval before new posts could be created.

Lack of authority over human resource management at tertiary hospitals was exacerbated in each country because certain staff were not accountable to the hospital or the MOH but looked to other ministries for promotion, leave and transfers. Ghana illustrates the general problem: specialists were employed by the University of Ghana Medical School and accountants by the Controller and Accountant General Department, often making them immune from or disinterested in the Chief Administrator's directions or wishes.

Financial management

Some degree of financial autonomy had been delegated to the case study organisations as compared to other hospitals in the country or the pre-autonomy situation. All the organisations were predominantly government-financed but received block grants for non-staff recurrent expenditure instead of stricter line item budgets. Again, hospitals in Thailand appeared to have the greatest level of freedom with a mixed system that gave complete control over a block grant component and considerable flexibility with other line items such as 'materials' (Bennett et al. 1998).

Authority to charge fees and flexibility over how fee revenue was spent increased financial autonomy substantially at Thai hospitals (50 per cent of expenditure), Ghana's teaching hospitals (20 per cent) and was a significant comparative management advantage for SJGH in Sri Lanka (30 per cent) since fees were not charged at other government hospitals. In Zimbabwe, Parirenyatwa held a similar comparative advantage at the time of the research due to its capacity to retain fee revenue.[1]

Procurement

Procurement regulations in all the countries specified that hospitals must purchase the bulk of their drugs and supplies from a government central medical stores. In Sri Lanka hospitals had to allocate 95 per cent of their medical supplies budget in this way but in Thailand the rules were less strict – at least 80 per cent of the drug budget had to go to the Government Pharmaceutical Organization (GPO), but these rules did not apply to user-fee revenue.

Freedom from political interference

A critical limit to any additional autonomy granted to an organisation was the degree to which the Minister used his or her prerogative in the legislation to issue directives and override board decisions. Four major areas where political imperatives often appeared to override managers' decisions were: the levels at which fees could be set, recruitment of senior consultants and other key personnel, capital expenditure, and the way block grant funds were allocated in practice. This was the case in the Ghanaian teaching hospitals, at Parirenyatwa in Zimbabwe, at APPVP in India and at SJGH in Sri Lanka. While it was appropriate that hospital boards were ultimately accountable to an elected Minister, the main problem in the case study countries appeared to be the norm of political interference in operational management decisions:

> It is a matter of debate as to whether we are autonomous or not. On paper yes, in practice my hands are tied by these politicians (Hospital Director, SJGH)

Hospital 'autonomy' policy in practice therefore represented a limited degree of decentralisation, rather than 'autonomisation' or the more radical 'corporatisation'. For example, in Ghana, it resembled deconcentration to the two tertiary hospitals rather than any form of delegation.

4.   Performance

Management structures, responsibilities and incentives had not radically changed for the hospitals in the five countries, so performance was unlikely to have changed. Indeed, assessment of policy impact was a minor part of the research since implementation had been delayed in Ghana and a national policy did not exist in Sri Lanka, India or Zimbabwe, making an assessment of performance before and after reform difficult or inappropriate. Nevertheless, evidence of performance sheds light on an organisation's capacity to provide services so where some autonomy had been implemented, basic data on performance were collected from the case study organisations using secondary sources and key informant interviews.

4.1   Resource mobilisation, service quality and the problem of equity

In Thailand and at SJGH, substantial user fee revenue facilitated rapid and flexible procurement of medical supplies and other inputs and recruitment of temporary staff, factors likely to improve quality of care and technical efficiency (Bennett et al. 1998; Russell and Attanayake 1997).

From a user perspective in Sri Lanka, the SJGH provided better services than a comparable, centrally managed hospital[2] with respect to cleanliness, politeness of staff, less overcrowding and shorter waiting times (Russell and Attanayake 1997). Interviews with managers at both hospitals suggested that SJGH could repair equipment and procure medical inputs faster because of its freedom to use fee revenue to purchase from the private sector when the need arose. In contrast, the other hospital experienced drug shortages more frequently than SJGH and these took longer to rectify because of stricter government procurement procedures.

The evaluation of the APVVP in India also identified resource mobilisation advantages and quality improvements associated with greater autonomy from bureaucratic regulations. Improvements were reported for water, toilet and electricity supply across the 162 hospitals and nearly half had had comprehensive buildings maintenance (Chawla and George 1996).

Freedom to charge fees and use revenue flexibly appeared to have led to service improvements at SJGH and at Thai hospitals, but the benefits of additional revenue raised an important question: is management autonomy necessary to improve services, or could this objective have been achieved within the old organisational set up simply with an injection of extra government resources? For example, in the cases of SJGH and APVVP, were better services the result of management autonomy *per se*, or the extra resources which greater autonomy facilitated? At the centrally managed hospital that was compared with SJGH, for example, lack of money was the main cause of drug and staff shortages and overcrowding.

4.2 Efficiency, effectiveness and innovation

There was limited evidence that autonomy led to improved technical efficiency. At SJGH, greater autonomy over spending probably led to better quality at higher cost. There was consensus amongst MOH staff and doctors at both hospitals that SJGH was a 'high cost' hospital compared to the centrally managed one. Expenditure per IP day comparisons suggested this opinion was correct (Table 4.3), and staff 'productivity' expressed as inpatient days per staff member was higher at the centrally managed hospital since it had fewer staff and a higher workload (Table 4.4). In addition, the centrally managed hospital used its bed capacity more efficiently with a bed occupancy rate of 93 per cent compared to 60–70 per cent at SJGH. No firm conclusions can be drawn, however, since the centrally managed hospital's lower costs and higher staff productivity might have reflected a slightly different case-mix or lower quality services caused by underfunding and thinly spread resources.

Improved efficiency from autonomy was most clearly evident at the TN Medical Supply Corporation. Prior to the formation of the TNMSC

Table 4.3   Comparison of expenditure per inpatient day (Rupees) at SJGH and a comparable centrally managed hospital in Sri Lanka, 1995

	SJGH	Centrally managed hospital
Salary cost per IP day	364	223
Total expenditure per IP day	947	405

Source: Russell and Attanayake, 1997.

Table 4.4   Staff productivity at SJGH and a comparable centrally managed hospital, 1995

	SJGH	Centrally managed hospital
Inpatient days per nurse	465	694
Inpatient days per doctor	1510	2529

Source: Russell and Attanayake, 1997.

in 1995, each hospital or district purchased drugs from suppliers at prices approved by the state Central Purchasing Committee. This piecemeal approach to purchasing prevented savings from bulk purchases, a large number of non-essential drugs were purchased, there was no quality control, and stocks were not recorded or controlled which often contributed to drug shortages. The TNMSC improved efficiency and effectiveness in the following ways (Bennett and Muraleedham 1998):

- it rationalised the drug list to 240 generic drugs;
- it introduced stricter quality control procedures;
- it obtained lower prices than the government because it was perceived to be a more timely and reliable payer;
- from the perspective of staff and patients, the quantity and quality of drug supply improved;
- there was improved needs assessment and better matching of supply with need;
- a sophisticated computer system was implemented linking each district drug store with the centre to monitor stocks and disbursements to facilities;
- in the first year of operation it saved Rs 380 million compared to the previous drug budget due to more efficient use of drugs and lower purchase prices.

Overall, two tentative conclusions emerge from the above analysis. First, greater autonomy to raise additional resources can potentially lead to better quality services. However this may have serious implications for equity of access since the greater the financial independence from the MOH, with reductions in central subsidies, the more hospitals will be forced to pursue cost recovery. Second, the fact that the most positive experience came from drug supply agencies (the TNMSC and also the State Pharmaceutical Corporation in Sri Lanka: Russell and Attanayake 1997) raises the question of whether 'autonomisation' might not be a more appropriate reform strategy for government drug supply agencies than for hospitals: drug purchasing and distribution are less complex tasks which are easier to specify and monitor.

5.   Capacity

Given limited hospital autonomy across the five countries, of more relevance than performance evaluation were explanations for why a policy of autonomy was not on the agenda in Sri Lanka and India, why implementation had been delayed or remained at an embryonic stage elsewhere, and what capacities were needed to take an autonomy policy forward.

5.1 Capacity to develop policy frameworks and initiate change

In Ghana in 1988, moving towards *full* self-financing through user fees was an overambitious and unrealistic goal. It was also doubtful whether the government really intended to delegate full hiring-and-firing authority to the hospitals at a time of increasing central control over the civil service payroll. There were no subsequent MOH policy documents setting out the respective roles of the MOH and the Boards and the practicalities for implementation, suggesting that neither the MOH nor the hospital management had a vision of what hospital autonomy might look like in practice:

> This put the Boards in a 'double-bind'. On the one hand, the MOH argued that the Board and management should take the lead in developing proposals for implementing autonomy. On the other hand, the MOH had not given guidance on what it was looking for. (Smithson, Asamoa-Baah and Mills 1997: 41)

Inattention to detail and implementation strategy also suggested that the law contained more political rhetoric than commitment to decentralisation. The political context in which Law 209 was introduced strengthened this argument, since it was passed by a highly centralised and undemocratic regime which had seized power by force (Ayee 1997). However, the more recent Ghana Health Service and Teaching Hospitals Act of 1996 set out legal frameworks more clearly and was complemented with detailed MOH plans to guide early phases of implementation, reflecting stronger commitment to reform and improved central MOH capacity to develop policy proposals and persuade other stakeholders that reform was feasible.

Whether decentralisation is driven by political or managerial objectives, it is implicitly a political process requiring shifts in political power and resource control. Central actors must be willing to cede decision-making powers which at the least requires them to have confidence in the hospital's financial management and accountability. Yet in Ghana in 1988, a variety of central stakeholders whose co-operation was required to implement the policy were not consulted. The PNDC Law 209 was passed by a government accustomed to legislation by decree through a top-down process which neglected consultation with the Public Services Commission, the Office of the Head of the Civil Service, the Ministry of Finance and the Controller and Accountant General. But without the support of the first two, hospitals could not break free from central control over staff management, while support from the latter two was necessary to shift from strict line budgets to a block grant.

Progress with hospital autonomy since 1995 stemmed from more concerted MOH efforts to develop new financial frameworks, set out the responsibilities of the MOH and the Board, and articulate this vision to key stakeholders. In 1994 the boards took the initiative and held consultative meetings with the central MOH and other key stakeholders which built consensus over frameworks and mechanisms for financial decentralisation, culminating in KBTH and KATH securing approval from the MOF and Controller and Accountant General to operate on a grant-funded basis in 1995 and 1996 respectively.

Resistance to decentralisation by central stakeholders was a major barrier to policy development in Zimbabwe, India and Sri Lanka. In Sri Lanka, central MOH and MOF actors used technical capacity constraints at sub-national levels, such as lack of accounting staff and management skills, to justify previous limited decentralisation. Senior MOH actors argued that these capacity constraints would lead to management failure if greater autonomy to tertiary hospitals were granted, and also emphasised the potential problem of corruption resulting from loss of central financial control:

> they do not have the facilities ... we would need to increase accounting staff and other cadre levels at teaching hospitals ... but cadre approval from the Treasury would be needed and the resources are not there. We would also give up our control of these hospitals and they are big spenders!
> ... they lack skills, accountants and we would get corrupt things going on ... how could we keep track of what they are spending?

These technical arguments were nevertheless located within a wider political and institutional context antagonistic to decentralisation: a bureaucratic structure and management culture based on central control; the MOH, which historically had been unwilling to decentralise; and a widespread assumption amongst central state actors that decentralisation inevitably led to financial irregularities lower down the system. In Ghana, Zimbabwe, India and Thailand, similar institutional barriers to decentralisation were identified. It is also likely in all countries that central actors themselves benefited from the rent-seeking opportunities created by centralised control over resources: in Thailand, for example, an active media has exposed on a number of occasions the personal benefits derived by politicians and senior civil servants from influencing the placing of large contracts.

5.2 MOH capacity to implement autonomy

Management weaknesses at sub-national levels may have been a genuine concern for central MOH actors, but it can be argued that the main stumbling block lay at the centre (or at state level in India) which had the responsibility to develop policy, manage the transition towards decen-tralised management and improve management systems and skills at lower levels. Strengthened management capacity at sub-national levels is at least in part dependent on the implementation of a decentralised system which gives managers the opportunity to use new systems and skills and learn from experience.

Decentralising management control to hospitals necessitates a new form of financial accountability between the Board and the central MOH, founded on good accounting systems and an information system that collects basic data on service outputs. If contracts and performance measurement tools are introduced, a more advanced financial informa-tion system which enables managers to scrutinise costs, set prices and monitor performance requires development.

Systems

In the case study countries, accounting systems within the existing bureaucratic set-up were designed for central financial control and were not management-oriented. They often functioned poorly: for example, routine accounting systems in Zimbabwe were failing to provide accurate or timely accounts for different cost centres due to inadequate staffing and low morale. In contrast, in Thailand, routine accounting and administra-tion systems were operational and generally reliable (Bennett et al. 1998).

These problems suggested that efforts to strengthen basic accounting and other administrative and human resource systems were critical regardless of the stage of reform, and were certainly a precondition for the development of financial information systems which could measure costs. This was the approach taken in Zimbabwe and Ghana, where efforts to improve accounting and general management systems and skills were supported by bilateral and multilateral donors (see Box 4.1).

Box 4.1   Developing financial information systems in Zimbabwe

The ODA's Health Management Strengthening Project (1991-95) placed a Technical Co-operation Officer for Financial Planning and Management at the MOHCW in 1992. Several weaknesses with the accounting system were identified on arrival: it was highly centralised with no local ownership of accounts, reducing incentives to keep accurate accounts and preventing facility managers from accessing accurate accounts information. The system did not link financial inputs with activities so did not produce data that allowed managers to monitor the efficiency of resource use.

A first step was to improve the accountancy regime since any improvement to financial planning and management was dependent on the availability of relevant and reliable data (Grant and Beach 1994: 9). Since 1992 the system has been decentralised to over 57 cost centres (central and provincial hospitals and districts), with each cost centre responsible for its own accounting. This brings benefits of ownership and local knowledge of account status, and managers can purchase items with greater knowledge of resource consequences.

The next step was the staged introduction, of a computerised financial management system, first at the five central hospitals then at the eight provincial offices. The system aimed to produce a management report each month for each cost centre, which included cost per inpatient day, cost per OP or IP and tables comparing costs across districts. Implementation was slow because it was not owned or driven by wider government reform of accounting and management systems.

Skills, incentives and motivation

Improved systems must be complemented by the skills and motivation to use them. In the core case study countries, the skills required to perform basic accounting procedures existed but low motivation amongst accountants, described in Zimbabwe as 'over stretched, poorly paid with no career prospects', meant slow and incomplete data returns from the bottom of the system upwards. Consequently, in Zimbabwe, implementation of the new financial management system was slow. In addition, incentives to change accounting procedures were limited because the new system was optional – there was no directive from the Ministry of Finance to force its use. Instead there were a few individuals within the MOHCW whose job it was to upgrade the accounting system and implement the financial management system. Meanwhile, MOHCW clerks had to continue to operate within the old accounting system. One MOHCW informant summarised these problems:

> We are trying to develop and implement a new system at the MOHCW which is not part of any government directive, so people are not driven to do the work. As soon as you walk away from a department at the central hospital or from the PMD's office, the staff often revert to what they were doing before. You cannot blame them for this – they must still comply with old procedures.... The challenge was to get them ready for proper income and expenditure accounting but to stay within the Treasury system.

The two key problems of centralised accounting systems and limited staff motivation to invest in or use new information systems strongly indicate that progress with decentralisation requires support from other Ministries and wider reform of public sector institutions.

5.3   The wider policy environment

While major stumbling blocks for reform were capacity constraints within Ministries of Health, the binding constraint in each country appeared to be the wider institutional and political environment. The main actors or contexts which had an impact on the reform process are mapped in Figure 4.1. Since these external capacity constraints recur across the different chapters and are summarised in Chapter 8, they are elaborated on below only where there are issues specific to autonomy or to particular countries.

Public sector institutions

Because the MOH is embedded within wider public sector regulations, it cannot unilaterally decide to introduce new accounting systems, delegate powers to hire and fire, increase fee levels or move to grant-based funding. Progress with increasing the degrees and functions of autonomy requires overarching reforms of public sector institutions controlled by powerful agencies at the apex of the state apparatus, including the Ministry of Finance and the Public Service Commission. Strong political backing and public support are also necessary to push reforms through since the changes envisaged are likely to threaten the interests and power of these state agencies.

Public sector trade union opposition to hospital autonomy was and will continue to be an institutional barrier to policy development in all the case study countries, but particularly in Zimbabwe and Sri Lanka, largely

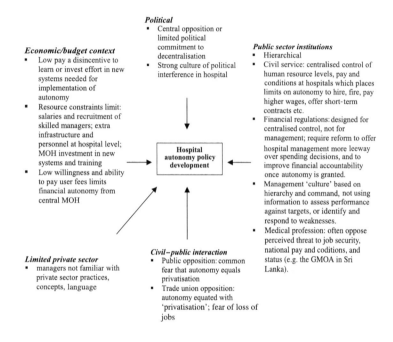

Figure 4.1 Constraints to policy development: the political, institutional and economic environment

because it was construed as privatisation and perceived as a threat to job security, wages and other public sector fringe benefits.

A key policy actor was the medical profession, which was supportive of greater autonomy in Ghana but very cautious in Sri Lanka. In Sri Lanka the Government Medical Officers Association (GMOA) had opposed decentralisation in the past: for example, in 1988, doctors had refused to be placed under the control of newly created Provincial Councils largely because of the prestige of being 'All Island' public servants and the perceived benefits of a national system of salaries and scales. A similar issue was evident in Andhra Pradesh where doctors had fears about job security following the creation of APVVP.

A sensitisation workshop on hospital autonomy in Sri Lanka which aimed to stimulate discussion and elicit the views of hospital managers, MOH officials and representatives of the GMOA found very little support for the concept of hospital autonomy, for the following reasons:

- There was a consensus that an effective national health service was in place and that 'autonomy' may threaten this system. Instead there was perceived potential for a greater degree of authority for some functions, for example increasing tender board thresholds or the amounts that could be shifted across budget headings.
- Autonomy was generally viewed as a structural transformation driven more by belief than evidence or common sense and would represent 'implementation of a failed system of autonomy from a developed country'. A more cautious reform process that first identified the strengths and weaknesses of the current system was advocated.
- SJGH was not viewed as a model for autonomy, mainly due to equity concerns. The main argument was that it was the role and obligation of government hospitals to ensure access to services and they could not turn patients away, whereas SJGH could do so to avoid the common 'floor patient'[3] problem. The hospital could only survive morally and politically because it was an exception within a national system that provided services free at the point of delivery. As there were several other tertiary hospitals which provided free services, SJGH could pursue a substantial level of cost recovery without threatening equity or the political principle of free health care.
- Caution against any form of decentralisation was reinforced by problems which had been experienced with devolution to provinces after 1988. This had extracted provincial and base hospitals from the central line Ministry and placed them under the control of provincial councils. In practice this had added another layer of politicians and increased political interference and restrictions on hospital management. Provincial hospital managers wanted to be free from provincial council control and taken back under the central line ministry. Paradoxically, this process of recentralisation is now taking place to give hospital managers more flexibility and autonomy.

Across the case study countries, public sector management styles and cultures posed constraints to the development of the new accounting and financial information systems required to facilitate accountability within a decentralised system. There was widespread indifference to information as a management tool, and the absence of an information orientated management culture, a product of past management practices based on hierarchy, command and duty. At all levels of the system, changing people's perceptions about the importance of information and attitudes towards data analysis as a tool would be a long-term process:

Even if you had the new system up and running, people's capacity to internalise change, to start thinking and operating in a new way with a new system, is limited ... these things take time wherever change is introduced (MOHCW informant).

Political caution about reform

Political opposition to decentralisation, or at least a situation of political inertia, was strongest in Sri Lanka and India. In Sri Lanka, senior politicians were reluctant to advocate any reform of hospital management which offered only abstract benefits but concrete political risks, particularly at central hospitals which had a high political profile especially when problems arose. In Sri Lanka there also remained a widespread perception that the state's role was to directly provide health services free at the point of delivery for the benefit of the poor and other sections of society (Russell and Attanayake 1997; Silva, Russell and Rakodi 1997). Opposition to a policy of autonomisation was likely to be widespread and vociferous, mobilised by trade unions, left-wing political organisations and whichever political party happened to be in opposition.

Private sector development

Levels of private sector development can be important in influencing the pace and nature of reform. In countries with greater private sector development, a policy of autonomy may be easier to develop because: (a) there are more managers familiar with the tasks, skills and responsibilities of managing an autonomous organisation, and who are familiar with the associated language, concepts and practices, and (b) ideas about 'good management' and expectations of having to perform well are likely to be more prevalent. These potential benefits of a strong private sector were more available in Thailand than in the core case study countries. Moreover, relatively low public sector management salaries in the core case study countries encouraged good managers to move from the public to the private sector.

6.   Conclusions

6.1   Autonomy in reality

Hospital autonomy was not firmly on the policy agenda in India and Sri Lanka, only at proposal stage in Zimbabwe and Thailand, and at an early stage of implementation in Ghana. Autonomy, like decentralisation, varies in degree and in the functions it covers, and in practice changes were marginal. It is therefore difficult to draw even tentative conclusions about the impact of greater management autonomy on hospital performance.

Greater policy development in Africa might simply have reflected weaker government negotiating capacity and resilience to donors than in South Asia, and not widespread ideological or political commitment to reform. In South Asia, the economic crisis was not as deep-rooted, government service provision arrangements stronger and more stable, and donor leverage weaker. In Sri Lanka, many MOH officials were unfamiliar with the reform agenda, indifferent to it or opposed to it. In Thailand, an autonomous agency policy was being adopted by the government, but the exploration of its relevance to hospitals seems to have been the result of donor conditionality following the economic crisis in 1997 which resulted in social sector loans. The central MOH appeared to be at best lukewarm about increased hospital autonomy.

The pace of reform was also heavily influenced by factors within each country, in particular the degree of resistance to reform by bureaucratic and political actors at the centre, and the extent to which high-level MOH actors and medical professionals were pushing for change. Ghana may have been further down the path towards hospital autonomy than Sri Lanka because the MOH and medical profession were far more proactive, whereas in Sri Lanka these actors resisted reform. The particular direction of reform was also guided by the priorities of these policy actors: for example, Ghana had made more progress with hospital autonomy than Zimbabwe, but Zimbabwe more progress with contracting out.

Although hospital autonomy was extremely limited in all countries, it was a more common organisational arrangement for central government medical stores. In Tamil Nadu and Sri Lanka, medical stores had been granted corporate status and this had improved these organisations' effectiveness and efficiency (Bennett and Muraleedhan 1998; Russell and Attanayake 1997).

6.2 Capacity constraints and capacity development

Hospital autonomy in the form envisaged by the current NPM agenda represents a radical shift of responsibility to hospital managers and the possible use of contracts and performance agreements to promote transparency, accountability and performance. Slow progress with policy development can be ascribed to several dimensions of capacity, from narrow human resource and leadership weaknesses and weak information systems, to broader policy contexts such as centralised government institutions and management cultures and political resistance to reform.

The Ghana case illustrates the importance of capacity within the MOH organisation, in the form of skills and leadership, to develop clear and workable policy frameworks that can be placed before key stakeholders in the system. For example, alternative systems for human resource and financial management and new means of ensuring a hospital's financial accountability must be developed by the MOH. This requires the right technical and advocacy skills amongst a critical mass of MOH and hospital managers, and a leadership that can articulate ideas to different stakeholders. Leadership may be a critical factor: hospital autonomy is unlikely to work, even if formal rules are changed, without committed and competent leadership, for example, from a new team of managers brought in to transform the organisation and to push people to move away from old procedures and practices. Finally, even if the technical skills exist within the MOH, the medical profession as a whole must be supportive if change is to take place, as the contrasting situations in Ghana and Sri Lanka illustrated.

Broader dimensions of capacity, rooted in the overall history and development of government systems and institutions, are a major constraint on policy development. The MOH cannot grant critical dimensions or degrees of autonomy unilaterally or at the stroke of a pen. Change must first take place at the highest levels of government, which raises serious questions about the possibility of reform if efforts are focused on the health sector alone. Again in Ghana, the MOH showed some capacity to pursue broader changes by achieving concessions from the Ministry of Finance.

Due to the capacity constraints identified, policy development is likely to be gradual, starting with deconcentration rather than any form of autonomisation. Once accounting and reporting procedures are performed well enough for a block grant system to be managed effectively, further steps towards autonomy may be feasible. Capacity strengthening is therefore also likely to be gradual and to focus first on routine administrative functions, as was the case in Ghana:

> Over the last eight years, there has been significant investment in strengthening the government's capacity to manage the health sector. Some of the language has been consistent with the 'new' role of government but much of the effort has been devoted to strengthening the traditional task of government, by strengthening internal planning and management systems. (Smithson, Asamoa-Baah and Mills 1997: vii)

Capacity strengthening is likely to be not only gradual but iterative. Once a degree of decentralisation has taken place and hospital staff have the opportunity to use and learn new systems and skills, there will be stronger systems and a pool of experienced staff in place which will be able to cope with greater degrees of decentralisation. Three key phasing and capacity building questions will then arise. Which dimensions and degrees of decentralisation will be most useful to managers? Which will best develop their capacity for greater decentralisation in the future? And which will place the least demand on capacity and can be undertaken first? However, the fundamental issue of the extent to which public hospitals should be given greater autonomy, or indeed corporatised, remains very much an open question, and one which deserves much greater attention.

5
Increasing Government Finance: Charging the Users

1. Introduction

Like the other reforms examined in this book, a policy of user fees necessitates a degree of decentralisation and new management capacity. But, on an *a priori* basis, such a policy can be expected to be less demanding on government capacity than contracting out, or regulation and enablement of the private sector, since they require no radical organisational restructuring, no changes in the public private delivery mix, nor a shift from direct to indirect service provision roles. Nevertheless, it is well recognised that effective implementation of user-fee policy requires government capacity to perform effectively a range of routine collection, accounting and administrative functions, as well as new financial management roles at central and sub-national levels, and the most difficult task of the effective implementation of exemptions targeted at the poor and vulnerable (Gilson, Russell and Buse 1995).

This chapter begins with an overview of user-fee policy rationales, and the complementary contexts and government capacities that past research has shown to be necessary for policy success. The forces explaining the absence of user fees in Sri Lanka and India, and their implementation in Ghana, Zimbabwe and Thailand, are reviewed in section 2. User-fee policy experience in the latter three countries is then analysed, starting with a summary of policy performance in section 4 to shed light on government capacity to perform policy roles. Section 5 seeks to explain performance or impact by examining different aspects of government capacity affecting the design and implementation of user-fee policy. Where relevant, the Kenyan experience of user fee policy implementation, documented in Collins et al. (1996), is also drawn upon to shed light on how implementation strategy and capacity influence policy impact. Section 6 draws conclusions and highlights key issues relating to the implementation of user fee policy that arise from the study.

2. User-fee policies: why and how?

Two broad categories of user-fee system have been identified through reviews of user-fee experience: national user fee systems implemented at tertiary, secondary and primary levels throughout the country; and community financing initiatives at primary and peripheral levels of the health system, often supported and coordinated at national level (Bennett and Ngalanda-Banda 1994; Gilson 1997; Nolan and Turbat 1995). The objectives of the two systems differ slightly, with community financing in particular focusing on the sustainability of primary health care, assured essential drugs and decentralised decision-making in which communities play an active role (Jarrett and Ofosu-Amaah 1992). In general, both systems implicitly aim to tackle problems of sustainability in the health system through revenue generation to improve health service provision (Gilson 1997).

Analysts and donors also advocate national user-fee systems as a means of addressing inefficiencies and inequalities in the health system (Griffin 1992; Shaw and Griffin 1995; World Bank 1987 and 1993). Efficiency gains can, in theory, be derived from a cascading fee system which promotes better use of the referral system, and if fee revenue is used to address input shortages and improve the quality and utilisation of primary care facilities. The equity benefits of fees, by far the more contentious assertion, can be achieved if revenue is reallocated and targeted to poorer and under-served sections of society, and if an effective exemption system to protect the poor is implemented.

In other words, national user-fee systems, which are the focus of this chapter, have been justified on the grounds that they can strengthen the quality, efficiency and equity of the health system as a whole. However, previous research has shown that achievement of these objectives is critically dependent upon supportive policy contexts and policy measures, and government capacity to implement policy effectively (Bennett, Russell and Mills 1996; Gilson 1997; Gilson, Russell and Buse 1995; Kutzin 1995; Nolan and Turbat 1995). The following appear to be the most critical:

- decentralised revenue retention to provide incentives to collect fees and allow local quality improvements;

- accounting, auditing and financial management information systems which support management at all levels;
- financial management skills, especially at sub-national levels where revenue is managed;
- well-motivated staff with balanced financial incentives that encourage the adoption of new charging and management practices, but discourage overzealous or illegal charging;
- a well-designed and appropriate exemption system, with information that permits the target group to be reached;
- central leadership, training and guidance on exemption policy implementation and use of revenue;
- maintenance of government funding levels to ensure that fee revenue is additional and can be used for quality improvements and improved staff motivation;
- public willingness and ability to pay.

These conclusions from the literature provided the backdrop to the design of the research on user fee policy in the case study countries.

3.   User-fee policy and practice

3.1   Resisting reform in South Asia

While user fees were an integral component of structural adjustment programmes in Zimbabwe, Ghana and many other Sub-Saharan African countries, this was not the case in Sri Lanka, Tamil Nadu, India in general or other South Asian countries. In Sri Lanka, 20 years of economic liberalisation had not been accompanied by 'adjustment' in government social sectors, with user fees and other health sector reform initiatives excluded from the policy agenda. Whilst a few academics and consultants had advocated user fees and decentralised revenue retention (Ernst and Young 1994; Griffin, Levine and Eakin 1994; Wanasinghe 1994), their voice was weak in the face of widespread opposition to fees that harnessed an embedded and powerful discourse favourable to direct health (and other social) service delivery free at the point of delivery. Historically, Sri Lankan development policy had had a strong commitment to redistribution with growth, and direct service delivery (Drèze and Sen 1989). Indeed, since the 1930s, public action and state responses had politically and socially constructed health care as a public good, a basic right for all citizens (Sen 1988). Thus a high level Presidential Task Force for health care policy stated:

The commitment to provide comprehensive promotive, preventive, curative and rehabilitative health care, free at the point of delivery and within easy access to the entire populations, has been the fundamental premise on which successive governments based actions for meeting the needs of the people. (Presidential Task Force 1992: 6)

The recently formulated government National Health Policy statement re-emphasised this commitment to free care:

The Government will remain committed to providing basic health care free of cost to the individual at the point of delivery, in State sector institutions. (Republic of Sri Lanka 1996: 4)

Indeed, opposition to fees was widespread and cut across social groups, including wealthier sections of society that still resorted to government inpatient services as they were perceived to be the best and most reliable. Moreover, these groups were cautious about fees due to fears of social tension and violence should they be introduced (Silva, Russell and Rakodi 1997).

Within this historical, social and political context, key policy actors opposed fees or were given little room for manoeuvre. These key actors included:

- trade unions, student organisations and radical left-wing groups that opposed fees;
- top politicians and bureaucrats, who feared the electoral consequences of introducing fees and a strong political backlash which could lead to a replay of the political violence experienced in the late 1980s;
- health professionals, managers and unions who supported free government care for the poor on equity grounds and encouraged private sector provision for those willing and able to pay.

MOH respondents also pointed to organisational and institutional barriers to user fees. Current financial regulations would not permit the MOH to retain revenue and even if this could be negotiated, fees might not be translated into service improvements due to weak management at lower levels and incentives for corruption. But the most serious capacity weakness preventing user fees was, in their opinion, the lack of information or administrative systems in place to target the poor effectively: 'if this problem could be overcome the political opposition to fees would be considerably reduced' (MOH official).

The situation was not dissimilar in India. The World Bank was exerting pressure for fees at the centre but its influence on policy was limited since it was at the state level that legislation had to be passed and policy implemented (Bennett and Muraleedharan 1998). There was also wide-spread acceptance that government services were mainly utilised by the poor which weakened the case for fees, especially at the primary level, and the widespread practice of informal charging meant many health workers opposed a formal user-fee system that would have reduce their access to the cash collected. Service quality may also have been too poor for fees to be a real option.

3.2.   User fees in Africa

In Sub-Saharan Africa, internal and external pressure to introduce user fees was stronger and civic opposition to such reforms weaker. In Ghana and Zimbabwe, the economic crises preceding stabilisation and adjust-ment were more severe than in Sri Lanka or India. In Zimbabwe real MOH expenditure fell by 14 per cent between 1990/1 and 1991/2, and in the following year by a further 29 per cent (Russell and Gilson 1997). Similarly, in Ghana, real government health spending in 1983 was only 20 per cent of its level in 1975 and fees were advocated by doctors and managers to maintain professional expectations of service standards:

> In Ghana the initial impetus for a radical revision of fees came from the MOH where acute shortages of commodities were the most visible result of the financial crisis. At one stage, the shortage of foreign exchange was such that no drugs or medical supplies were imported for an entire year. (Smithson, Asamoa-Baah and Mills 1997: 22)

A reluctant government finally relented to pressure from the Ministry of Finance, MOH managers and medical professionals and increased fees in 1985. In Zimbabwe too there was internal pressure from the Ministry of Finance, some MOH officials and medical professionals to strengthen cost recovery, especially since the precedent had already been set by the Ministry of Education which had implemented fees in 1985.

Economic stagnation, foreign debt and deterioration of public services also increased susceptibility to donor pressure during the 1980s (Nolan and Turbat 1995; Russell and Gilson 1995), but this pressure varied from country to country. In Ghana pressure for cost recovery from the World Bank or IMF was limited, although these actors were not aloof from policy and endorsed fee increases in 1985, urging the government to recover 15 per cent of recurrent costs. In 1988 the World Bank injected financial resources into the influential 'cash and carry' revolving drug fund, which aimed to achieve full cost recovery from drug sales (Smithson, Asamoa-Baah and Mills 1997). In Zimbabwe, external pressure from the World Bank to increase fees was greater and fee increases were an integral component of the first structural adjustment programme in 1991.

Opposition to fees was limited or not effectively mobilised in Ghana and Zimbabwe, possibly because people were already paying informal charges at government facilities or resorting to the private sector, and because there were fewer channels to voice opposition and affect the policy (on Ghana, see Herbst 1993). While democratic institutions were far from perfect in Sri Lanka or Tamil Nadu, voters could at least remove an unpopular government. In contrast in Zimbabwe and Ghana, one-party politics and more limited democratic accountability meant politicians were less fearful of an electoral backlash or the 'political suicide' associated with fees in South Asia.

Nevertheless the governments of Ghana and Zimbabwe could neither ignore public sentiment nor the basic reality of affordability for the majority, so prices were set well below cost recovery levels. In Ghana, the populist regime tempered fee levels: for example, a major operation was set at 1,000 cedis instead of the 10,000 cedis recommended by the MOH, and in other cases MOH-recommended fee levels were halved to bring them to a level judged to be affordable to the average Ghanaian (Smithson, Asamoa-Baah and Mills 1997).

3.3 The Thai case

Unlike many other Asian and African states, Thailand had never provided health services for all, free at the point of delivery (Bennett et al. 1998). Around the turn of the century, hospitals collected revenue on a charitable basis: users were asked to contribute to the cost of their care in a donation box. Over the years this system gradually became formalised. Around 1937, a government health policy statement decreed that all those who could afford it should pay some part of the cost of their drugs. In many countries with colonial regimes, fees were repealed at independence, but Thailand was never part of a colonial power, and a desire to demonstrate commitment to social service provision for all never led to a reversal of the policy of charging for health care services. Furthermore, Thai culture was conducive to paying something for services received, and there never seems to have been resistance to contributing to the cost of care. Difficulties in payment and concern for the poor were addressed by specific selective schemes, rather than through comprehensive subsidies to all.

4.   Performance

This section provides an overview of policy outputs in Ghana, Zimbabwe and Thailand in order to shed light on government capacity to perform user-fee policy roles.

4.1   Revenue and sustainability

Cross-country reviews show that national user fee systems, on average, generate only 5 per cent of government recurrent health expenditure (Gilson, Russell and Buse 1995; Nolan and Turbat 1995). In Ghana policy had been quite successful in generating additional funding, the policy's main objective, with cost recovery ratios consistently above this average of 5 per cent, indeed reaching a maximum of 12.4 per cent in 1987, and as high as 20 per cent at the two main teaching hospitals (Smithson, Asamoa-Baah and Mills 1997). Implementation of the cash-and-carry revolving drug fund in 1993 increased national cost recovery ratios, with drug sales accounting for about 80 per cent of revenue.

Revenue generation had been less successful in Zimbabwe, with cost recovery ratios consistently below 3 per cent. Cost recovery strengthening in 1991 produced only a small increase in the cost recovery ratio, to 3.5 per cent, and it subsequently remained low even after fee increases in 1994, due to low prices and weak billing and collection systems. Thailand was more successful in terms of revenue generation, and at hospital level fee revenue made up about 50 per cent of total recurrent expenditure. This better performance stemmed from higher prices, partly made possible by exemption schemes, and combined with a more effective collection system which secured insurance reimbursements from patients covered by a variety of health insurance schemes, notably the Civil Service Medical Benefit Scheme for government employees (Tangcharoensathien, Supachutikul and Nitayarumphong 1992).

Comparison with non-staff recurrent expenditure at hospital level may provide a better indicator of user-fee revenue impact since it indicates the size of the extra cash resources at facility managers' disposal to spend on inputs. In Ghana, where a considerable proportion of government resources was centrally allocated and out of the hands of facility managers (payroll, medical supplies), user-fee revenue was often double the value of centrally allocated funds (Smithson, Asamoa-Baah and Mills 1997). In Thailand, fee revenue was even more important at hospitals, making up 80–90 per cent of non-staff recurrent expenditure (Bennett et al. 1998). In contrast in Zimbabwe, fee revenue had made no impact on facility managers' access to extra resources because all revenue was returned to the Treasury at the time of the research.

While user fees generated substantial revenue for the health sector in Ghana, an important question was whether these gains were neutralised by a corresponding reduction in government financing. While there is a counterfactual problem in assessing this (it is not known what would have happened if fees had not been introduced), there was some evidence to suggest this may have been the case (Smithson, Asamoa-Baah and Mills 1997), implying that fee revenue was not used to improve quality but rather to sustain services which might otherwise have failed due to input shortages, particularly at the primary level.

In Zimbabwe, fee revenue had not compensated for large reductions in government health spending, which by 1995/6 was 40 per cent below its 1990 level in terms of its real value per capita. The real value of the government's drug purchase fund had also dropped by 20 per cent in the first two years of structural adjustment, and in per capita terms drug spending fell by one-third between 1990 and 1995. Real spending on salaries also fell by one-third between 1990 and 1995, leading to a continuing exodus of health workers to the private sector or abroad (Watkins, forthcoming).

4.2 Revenue use, quality and technical efficiency

Before the drug 'cash and carry' system was introduced in Ghana, drug supplies were scarce, erratic and a major cause of public discontent with government health services. The 'cash and carry' system resulted in better service quality with respect to drug availability and, possibly, improved technical efficiency. However, fees may have reduced efficiency due to resulting drops in utilisation; charges were not cascaded downwards to encourage appropriate use of the referral system; and perverse incentives for inappropriate or over-prescribing also existed (Smithson, Asamoa-Baah and Mills 1997).

In Zimbabwe, the impact of fees on quality was difficult to judge but was probably insubstantial because revenue was not retained by the health sector and fees were implemented at a time of deepening financial and human resource constraints. In focus group discussions, urban service users complained about basic service quality problems including drug shortages, rude staff and long waiting times, which had persisted despite higher charges (Mutizwa-Mangiza 1997).

4.3 Utilisation and equity

User-fee policy can, in theory, promote equity objectives if exemptions for the poor or vulnerable are included but in all three countries this is where policy was weakest and most heavily criticised. In the Volta region of

Ghana, fees led to a 50 per cent drop in outpatient attendances, a trend that was later reversed in urban but not rural areas, suggesting the rural poor were disproportionately affected (Waddington and Enyimayew 1989; 1990). Qualitative evidence also showed that fees imposed barriers to access or large financial burdens on the poor (Korboe 1995; Norton et al. 1995), a problem exacerbated by people's uncertainty about prices caused by local and illegal charging practices.

In Zimbabwe, the negative utilisation impact of fees was less dramatic, probably because prices were lower and collection not as strictly enforced as in Ghana. Utilisation levels had, none the less, declined, especially for antenatal care and length of stay in maternity wards (Hongoro and Chandiwana 1993), and there was also substantial qualitative data showing affordability problems (Lennock 1994; Mutizwa-Mangiza 1997):

> Low income residents in the three cities made it clear that they do not normally budget for health expenses... If an illness occurs in the family, money is diverted from food, rent, school fees or water. (Mutizwa-Mangiza 1997: 21)

> In interviews, doctors mentioned that a large number of patients refuse certain investigations and procedures, in an attempt to reduce the hospital bill. They also described many instances of patients who they had discharged with a prescription, but who then came back worse off because they had been unable to procure the drugs because of financial constraints. (Mutizwa-Mangiza 1997: 17)

This aspect of user-fee policy impact underlines concern about the policy's appropriateness in contexts of rural and urban poverty, where revenue generation is likely to be low and where the financial burden placed on poor households may cause further impoverishment (Booth et al. 1995; Ensor and San 1996; Gilson, Russell and Buse 1995; Russell 1996).

5.   Capacity

This section identifies the different aspects of capacity which explain implementation difficulties and impact. Capacity constraints within the MOH organisation, related to weak systems, skills and incentives, were part of the problem. But the MOH and its staff were embedded within wider contexts and government structures and systems, and capacity problems within the MOH organisation stemmed from deficiencies within this broader incentive and policy environment. This broader policy environment is the starting point for analysis below, since it simultaneously drove user fee policy but weakened MOH capacity to subsequently design and implement it.

5.1   The policy environment and early policy processes

User-fee policies in Ghana and Zimbabwe were implemented when government capacity in general had been weakened. The government organisational environment was plagued by economic crisis, harsh cuts in social sector spending and a weakened and demoralised government administration. Government capacity to perform basic or routine administrative roles, such as maintaining accounts, preparing annual budget estimates or making timely payments to its workforce and suppliers, was limited or at the point of collapse. In such contexts, government capacity to perform new fee policy roles was likely to be extremely weak. In contrast in Thailand, fee and exemption systems were operating within a stronger economy and government bureaucracy.

Weakened government capacity to prepare for implementation was exacerbated by the speed with which fee policy was introduced in response to economic crisis. This lack of planning or capacity strengthening prior to implementation was not a surprising feature of the policy process however, given the delicate economic, political and administrative environment in which governments found themselves at the time of reform. In Ghana, for example, the government had to seize a window of political opportunity in 1985 so its strategy was to legislate first and worry about implementation later:

> The collapse of the government system at that time would have made it very difficult to implement a policy at all if the plan had been to strengthen capacity prior to policy implementation. (Smithson, Asamoa-Baah and Mills 1997: 33)

This absence of an implementation strategy, which could have involved a phased approach with capacity building, increased the likelihood of policy failure. This was highlighted in Kenya by Collins et al. (1996) where two different approaches to implementation were used. The first attempt, in late 1989, which was also driven by harsh economic conditions, was rushed, lacked strategy and allowed no time for staff training or testing of systems. As a result, implementation problems and policy failures arose, with cost recovery levels similar to Zimbabwe's (at about 3 per cent), no improvements in service quality and a dramatic 50 per cent decline in utilisation. Explanations for Kenya's early policy failures probably apply to Ghana and Zimbabwe as well:

> The initial implementation of cost sharing simultaneously at all facilities did not permit testing of fees and systems, proper training of staff, or adequate supervision. As a result implementation was weak and when problems emerged they were so widespread that the MOH was unable to take corrective action. (Collins et al. 1996)

The policy was implemented again in 1991 with USAID support, using a phased strategy to facilitate capacity strengthening over 3–4 years (see Box 5.1). A cascading approach was used to implement new collection, accounting and management systems and fee increases, starting with Kenyatta National Hospital, then the seven provincial hospitals, and so on downwards. Emphasis was placed on exploiting the biggest revenue

---

Box 5.1   Kenya's re-implementation strategy

Phase 1: Development of new management systems (1991–3): design of improved collection/exemption, spending procedures and accounting systems; introduction of systems through focused workshops; subsequent monthly supervision of each facility; systems cascaded down from provincial hospitals to district and then sub-district hospitals. Use of operations manuals which served as a constant reference point during training and implementation.

Phase 2: Increasing the acceptability of fees (1992–3): low outpatient fees reintroduced and impact monitored. Revenues increased by focusing on high revenue generating areas, in particular speeding up claims procedures for NHIF reimbursements at hospitals. Focus on using revenue to improve most visible aspects of quality.

Phase 3: Fee adjustments (1993–4): gradual increases in outpatient and inpatient fees, assessing patient and provider reactions.

Phase 4: Improved accountability (1993–4): through intensified supervision and monitoring; increased use of government disciplinary procedures; and establishment of district health management boards in 1992, which received training and began to play their role of approving expenditure plans and monitoring performance.

Source: Collins et al. (1996).

sources; in particular, National Hospital Insurance Fund (NHIF) claims were speeded up at hospitals.

Overall, this approach gave time to develop and test systems, train staff and generate experience higher up which could subsequently be harnessed for training at lower levels. It led to increased cost recovery – for example, 10 per cent at provincial hospitals and 6 per cent at district hospitals (Collins et al. 1996), and the burden of improved fee collection may have been disproportionately low for the poor because much of the increase in revenue at hospitals stemmed from NHIF claims, although the equity impact of fees remained unclear.

Another important component of implementation strategy lacking in Ghana and Zimbabwe was an information campaign for the public and health staff. This could have provided a stronger basis for subsequent implementation because patients would know whether they were eligible for exemption and what they would be charged, and staff would know their roles and understand why they were being asked to perform them. In Zimbabwe following the latest policy change in 1996 to allow revenue retention at facilities, district and provincial staff complained that they needed more information about user-fee retention and related rules and regulations, and guidance and training on how to spend the revenue. They argued that they could not implement the policy change without it.

5.2 Capacity to develop policy design

Because policy was driven largely by economic crises and resource shortages in the health sector, there was a narrow emphasis on raising revenue, and equity and efficiency objectives were given little priority. Consequently there were few policy mechanisms in place to reduce the burden of fees for poor households or to promote effective management of fee revenue. Indeed in Zimbabwe, cost recovery had few health sector objectives; it simply aimed to improve the fiscal balance and all revenue returned to the Treasury.

Policy design in both countries was flawed in several ways. With respect to fee schedules and the financial incentives they generated, several features seemed to be important. Provision for regular fee increases in line with inflation to sustain the revenue base were lacking in Ghana and Zimbabwe. In Ghana, drug prices were continuously revised in line with inflation but other service charges remained at levels specified in 1985 legislation[1] even though the value of fee levels had eroded by about 90 per cent since that date (Smithson, Asamoa-Baah and Mills 1997). Despite MOH demands, new legislation was not forthcoming due to political concerns.

These drastic declines in the real value of non-drug charges in Ghana generated strong incentives to increase fees with or without the tacit approval of the MOH; in other words, to levy illegal charges. Both practices caused wide and uncontrollable fee level discrepancies between facilities. Moreover, because drug sales were the main source of revenue for facilities in Ghana, there were strong financial incentives to over-charge or overprescribe to the detriment of the user (Smithson, Asamoa-Baah and Mills 1997). A key weakness of pricing policy was therefore the creation of financial incentives that did not balance revenue collection objectives with equity, efficiency and quality objectives.

Exemption policy design posed the greatest difficulties for policy-makers, due to the intractable difficulty of developing a targeting mechanism which effectively distinguished between patients who could and could not afford to pay. In each of the case study countries, the government, in its policy rhetoric, recognised that exemptions were critical and established eligibility criteria. For example, in Ghana, the law stated that 'paupers' or the 'destitute' should be exempt from fees. Unfortunately, the vagueness of these terms provided no guidance and left the decision to exempt wholly to the discretion of the facility health worker. And since these terms could easily be interpreted to mean only the most socially marginalised they did, in effect, classify the bulk of the poor as able to pay and ineligible for exemption.

In contrast, Zimbabwe and Thailand used specific income thresholds to define those eligible for exemption, but again these criteria were of limited use when systems were not in place to assess a patient's income. Income criteria were also inappropriate for large sections of the population which had in-kind or erratic incomes that defied systematic or accurate measurement.

Eligibility criteria also undermined exemption policy effectiveness in Ghana and Zimbabwe because 'non-poor' groups such as civil servants (including health workers) were included, causing loss of revenue. In Ghana, health workers were exempted from all fees under the 1985 regulations and were the biggest group to regularly receive exemption. Abuse of this system was eventually reduced by requiring health workers, along with other civil servants, to pay first and reclaim from their parent ministry. The result was a massive reduction in staff drug consumption.

A second problem with exemption policy design was the location of the screening procedure. In Ghana it appeared to be too decentralised with no national guidelines or checks and balances to ensure the poor were exempted across all facilities. In Zimbabwe the system was, in principle, less decentralised as discretion did not wholly lie at the facility level.

Patients could show a wage slip as written proof of their income status or, if they were unemployed, a letter obtained from the district office of the Department of Social Welfare (DOSW). But in practice this system was flawed because many people lacked wage slips or could not obtain the necessary letter from the DOSW, so the health worker had to decide whether to exempt from the patient's appearance and self-declared income. This decentralised system, when combined with the recent introduction of revenue retention, may have generated financial incentives in Zimbabwe not to exempt similar to those in Ghana.

Screening procedures in Thailand were also decentralised but received stronger central direction and guidance, and offered the poor the opportunity to seek exemption from two different sources: either the facility at the time of use or beforehand through screening in the community. In this latter approach, a Low Income Card (LIC) was allocated to households below a national income threshold, and identified by the village head and village committee which included a health volunteer. This system was potentially more accurate due to fewer information asymmetries at the village level compared to the facility; and it allowed an LIC holder to obtain free care automatically without having to be means-tested at each visit. It also reduced the incentives for the facility not to grant exemptions, since facilities received a special grant as recompense (although they complained it was inadequate to cover the value of the exemptions they gave).

The system was open to some abuse since the village head could dominate card allocation and the procedure was embedded in local social relationships and patron–client relations. However, it had been evaluated and strengthened over the previous 20 years and, from 1981, screening procedures were changed to address some of these problems. In the early 1990s, greater information dissemination to villagers, the inclusion of health volunteers in village committees and a more pro-active approach by the village committee to ensure that people applied led to an increase in LIC coverage from 7.6 million to 11 million people, with coverage of the target group increasing from 49 per cent to 80 per cent (Gilson et al. 1998).

While Thailand had made efforts to improve exemption targeting, in Ghana and Zimbabwe there had been no serious attempt to investigate or develop innovative exemption mechanisms. In Zimbabwe, for example, a senior MOHCW informant commented: 'We'll look at the exemption system later' (Russell et al. 1997).

Policy design in Ghana and Zimbabwe contributed to poor per-formance, especially with respect to equity, but the main difficulties lay with implementation and stemmed from capacity weaknesses within the MOH organisation and from the wider institutional and economic environment that was not supportive to policy implementation.

5.3   MOH organisational capacity to implement policy

A number of studies have found that the impact of fee systems is strongly influenced by organisational and managerial factors (Gilson 1997; Kutzin 1995; Mogedal, Steen and Mpelumbe 1995). As noted above, in Ghana and Zimbabwe MOH capacity to perform even routine administrative tasks was constrained by government-wide budget constraints and administrative capacity decline. MOH capacity to perform additional and new roles associated with user-fee and exemption policy implementation was, therefore, likely to have been extremely weak. In contrast in Thailand, there was no government-wide crisis at the time of the research and the MOH had over 20 years' experience of user-fee policy implementation. Necessary systems and skills for billing, fee collection and revenue use had been developed and the MOH proved reflective and adaptive by reforming the exemption system several times in response to evaluations that highlighted weaknesses (Bennett et al. 1998).

Organisational structures

Decentralised management structures are a basic capacity required for the effective implementation of user-fee policy. Without the authority to retain or use fee revenue, facility managers will have little incentive to collect fees and no capacity to improve services or develop experience with revenue management. In Zimbabwe, factors outside the control of the MOH meant this basic capacity was missing for the first five years of cost recovery (1991–6), contributing to low revenue collection.

Strengthening capacity at the centre to lead policy development and support sub-national levels is likely to require some form of organisational restructuring, for example, through a unit responsible for the design of new systems, operational guidelines, training and troubleshooting, or at least the clear allocation of responsibility for these tasks to existing units and staff. In Ghana following the introduction of fees, a unit devoted to policy implementation was not established due to the rushed policy process, resource shortages or possibly the absence of donor funds for capacity development.[2] The absence of a central 'policy champion' contributed to a long delay in the introduction of new reporting or accounting systems (until 1994) and lack of financial management training at all levels. The most frequently cited complaint at facility level was the lack of operational guidance, especially for spending revenue, which caused risk-averse managers to leave funds to accumulate in bank accounts, where their value was eroded by inflation. The absence of spending guidelines for the revolving drug fund contributed to spending on non drug items causing decapitalisation.

In Zimbabwe, no units or staff positions were established to develop and support fee and exemption policy. Following the more recent revenue retention policy, greater guidance and training was needed at sub-national levels. District and provincial level informants complained that they were still sending revenue to the Treasury because they had received no other instruction, or were saving the money until guidance arrived (Russell et al. 1997). Informants also argued that training in accounting and revenue management would be crucial to implementation:

> they [clerks] need to know about accounting procedures, what they can spend the money on ... most of our accounts staff have never actually done any expenditure planning ... (provincial official)

> for once these people will be dealing with real money, not figures on paper. They will need to set cost recovery objectives, decide on expenditure priorities ... Some basic training at our facilities is needed before we can start managing revenue ... even at provincial hospitals they will need support from the centre ... (central MOH official)

Systems, skills and motivation

Billing and collection systems: In Zimbabwe, two major factors undermining cost recovery were limited staff motivation to collect fees, and weak billing and collection systems (Hecht, Overholt and Homberg 1993). In central and provincial hospitals the billing system was cumbersome and too slow to cope with the workload as the clerk had to go to each department and manually prepare the bill. Patients often left the hospital before receiving a bill but even if a bill was provided, the patient could pay later by instalments, adding to the administrative burden. If payment was not forthcoming, the debt collection process was bureaucratic, time-consuming and often unsuccessful. In addition to systemic problems, MOH officials stated there were too few revenue clerks to deal with the patient workload and that they were inexperienced and lacked motivation due to low pay and limited promotion prospects (Russell et al. 1997).

In contrast in Ghana, there were strong incentives for health staff to collect fees (Gilson et al. 1995; Smithson, Asamoa-Baah and Mills 1997).

External aspects of capacity   **Internal aspects of capacity**

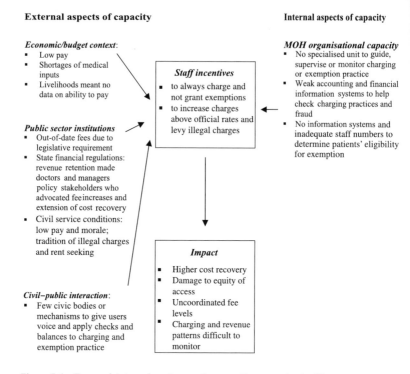

Figure 5.1   Forces driving charging and exemption practice in Ghana

This had a positive impact on cost recovery rates but also led to widespread local or illegal charging practices.

Exempting the poor: The way in which both external and internal capacity constraints came together to drive charging and exemption practices in Ghana is mapped out in Figure 5.1. Economic incentives to refuse exemptions for the poor were strong because fee revenue was a significant resource for facility staff and managers – they had become stakeholders in the system. Facility managers viewed exemptions as forgone income and a potential threat to the viability of the cash and carry revolving drug fund so there was no concerted effort to protect the poor (Smithson, Asamoa-Baah and Mills 1997). Weak implementation capacity at the facility, where responsibility lay for screening, compounded the problem. There were no information systems in place to help ascertain a person's income and staff shortages meant that many hospitals and almost all sub-district facilities lacked a social welfare officer.

In Zimbabwe, the incentives mapped out in Figure 5.1 were weaker. Facility managers, without access to the funds generated, were not yet stakeholders in the fee system. Nevertheless capacity weaknesses in the exemption system caused serious implementation problems which in turn led to access and payment difficulties for the poor (Kanji and Jazdowska 1993; Lennock 1994; Mutizwa-Mangiza 1997; Watkins, forthcoming). Scarcity of information about patients' income was a basic constraint, as in Ghana and other developing countries. Moreover the Social Development Fund (SDF)[3] set up by the government to finance exemptions was poorly planned and organised. The SDF did not become operational until 1992, over a year after cost recovery was strengthened; SDF resources were inadequate and could not meet the claims placed on it by different ministries; and there were basic administrative failures which prevented the eligible poor accessing exemptions (Mutizwa-Mangiza 1997; Russell et al. 1997; Watkins forthcoming):

- the DOSW screened exemption applicants but distance to the local DOSW office could be 40–100 km, posing insurmountable transport and time costs;
- application procedures were cumbersome and time-consuming, with documentation required to prove an income level below $Z400;
- no extra staff were recruited at DOSW offices, contributing to long queues; moreover this new task was added at a time when the DOSW budget fell by 26 per cent in real terms (Lennock 1994);
- approval of an exemption required final authorisation from the Harare office, increasing delays.

Exemption system capacity failures have been a basic flaw in user-fee policy in numerous countries (Booth et al. 1995; Gilson et al. 1995; Kanji and Jazdowska 1993; Russell 1996). Although the Thai example showed that exemption systems can be given greater priority and improved by governments, financial and administrative capacity weaknesses are likely to prevent Ghana and Zimbabwe from achieving similar results.

Accounting and financial information – systems, skills and incentives: the introduction of user fees demands more management-oriented accounting and financial information systems in Health Ministries. In Ghana and Zimbabwe, national government accounting systems and procedures were centralised, their main purpose being to control expenditure, and they did not supply useful information to managers such as revenue and spending patterns across cost centres. In both countries, routine accounting systems needed strengthening and new reporting systems were required to monitor revenue and spending patterns. These systems also required accompanying skills, primarily data analysis capabilities, and perhaps most importantly the responsibility and incentives to use them.

In Ghana, accounting systems were a constraint on better financial management and accountability. The introduction of standardised record books, vouchers and reporting forms did not take place until 1994, nine years after user fees had been increased. Inattention to the spending side was most vividly illustrated by the fact that facilities were not required to report on their use of revenue, and the information system was plagued by incomplete and inaccurate reporting with no possibility of analysing revenue or expenditure by cost centre (Smithson, Asamoa-Baah and Mills 1997). Zimbabwe may experience similar problems following revenue retention if new accounting systems are not developed and implemented.

Not only must the MOH develop new systems and train staff, it must also ensure that they are adopted and adhered to. In Ghana lack of supervision by regional and district accountants exacerbated non-compliance with new accounting and reporting procedures. Reporting remained patchy and was unlikely to improve until a combination of more interest and better supervision from managers at all levels was achieved (Smithson et al. 1997). Local charging practices made matters worse by loosening controls and making illegal charges and fraud more difficult to detect.

In both core case study countries, the MOH's ability to develop and implement new accounting, auditing and financial information systems was influenced by capacity within the MOH organisation itself. But disincentives to develop or comply with new systems also stemmed from the wider policy environment: Figure 5.2 maps out the internal and external constraints. For example, other ministries needed to be brought on board for new accounting systems to become operational, in particular the Ministry of Finance. If accountants and accounts clerks were not directed to adopt new systems by the Ministry of Finance and Accountant General's Office, they would have little incentive to do so.

5.4   Capacity: the wider policy environment

Capacity weaknesses within Ministries of Health in Ghana, Zimbabwe and Thailand were heavily influenced by wider public sector institutions and the political and economic environment. The broader contextual setting placed greater constraints on the Ministries of Health in the two African countries than in Thailand, because of greater resource constraints

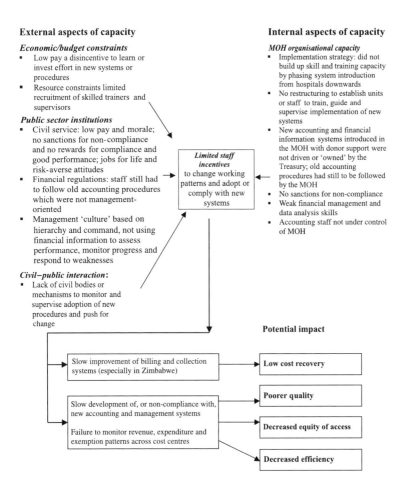

External aspects of capacity

Economic/budget constraints
- Low pay a disincentive to learn or invest effort in new systems or procedures
- Resource constraints limited recruitment of skilled trainers and supervisors

Public sector institutions
- Civil service: low pay and morale; no sanctions for non-compliance and no rewards for compliance and good performance; jobs for life and risk-averse attitudes
- Financial regulations: staff still had to follow old accounting procedures which were not management-oriented
- Management 'culture' based on hierarchy and command, not using financial information to assess performance, monitor progress and respond to weaknesses

Civil–public interaction:
- Lack of civil bodies or mechanisms to monitor and supervise adoption of new procedures and push for change

Internal aspects of capacity

MOH organisational capacity
- Implementation strategy: did not build up skill and training capacity by phasing system introduction from hospitals downwards
- No restructuring to establish units or staff to train, guide and supervise implementation of new systems
- New accounting and financial information systems introduced in the MOH with donor support were not driven or 'owned' by the Treasury; old accounting procedures had still to be followed by the MOH
- No sanctions for non-compliance
- Weak financial management and data analysis skills
- Accounting staff not under control of MOH

Limited staff incentives to change working patterns and adopt or comply with new systems

Potential impact

Slow improvement of billing and collection systems (especially in Zimbabwe)

Slow development of, or non-compliance with, new accounting and management systems

Failure to monitor revenue, expenditure and exemption patterns across cost centres

Low cost recovery

Poorer quality

Decreased equity of access

Decreased efficiency

Figure 5.2 Negative incentives in Zimbabwe and Ghana: capacity constraints on development of and compliance with new management systems and their potential impact

and because government administration was stronger and better functioning in Thailand. These 'external' aspects of capacity have already been used to explain the incentives and implementation problems which underlie policy performance in Figures 5.1 and 5.2.

This wider definition of capacity, which almost equates capacity with 'development' (Grindle and Hildebrand 1995), introduces more complex considerations of embedded bureaucratic structures, cultures and incentive problems that are rooted in government service more generally. These dimensions of capacity are less easily 'reformed'. In the case study countries these broader contexts affected:

- the prices that could be set, those eligible for exemption and those actually obtaining exemption. Dimensions of capacity included the political sensitivity of user fees; the lack of political voice and power of the poor vis-à-vis other sections of society; high levels of poverty and people's limited willingness and ability to pay; and the wider livelihood context which added to exemption policy difficulties;
- the MOH's capacity to change its accounting and management systems. Overarching financial regulations and procedures geared towards centralised control rather than devolved financial management were a deeply rooted institutional constraint to the development of new accounting and financial information systems and new attitudes towards the use of information for management purposes;
- the MOH's capacity to address pay and motivation problems. This was, to a large extent, outside of the MOH's control, since it was either a question of resources or Public Service Commission rules and regulations. Either the MOH had to be extracted from these constraints (for example, through the creation of an 'Executive Agency', which was proposed in Ghana) or the Public Service Commission tasks had first to be decentralised;
- the MOH's capacity to establish new units, develop new systems and begin training. The MOH was constrained by wider budget constraints and other government spending priorities, and by the more general motivation problems within government service.

6. Conclusions

User-fee policies, like other components of the health sector reform agenda, appear to be more advanced in Africa then South Asia on the basis of this and other research findings. In South Asia economic problems have been less severe, there has been less donor leverage and pressure, and internal forces for change in the public sector have been more limited, possibly because bureaucratic and political structures and vested interests are more established and stable (Cassels 1995).

Supportive policy contexts, policy measures and government capacities necessary for effective implementation of user fee policy were listed in section 2. All of these were absent or limited in Ghana and Zimbabwe but more evident in Thailand, which helps to explain why policy impact in the two African countries was less successful. In Zimbabwe, fees had a limited impact on revenue generation, efficiency and sustainability, and a detrimental impact on equity. In Ghana, stronger incentives to charge led to more success with revenue generation, particularly from drug sales, and allowed improvements to drug supplies and other service inputs. But cost-pricing for drugs and stricter fee collection probably caused more serious affordability and access problems than in Zimbabwe.

Three key issues relevant to future policy development arise from these case studies.

6.1 The importance of implementation strategy

The policy environment and capacity weaknesses in Ghana and Zimbabwe prevented planning or development of an implementation strategy. In Kenya, an implementation strategy was developed with strong support from the USAID-funded Kenya Health Care Financing Project. Several elements of this strategy appear to have had a significant impact. First, phasing allowed new accounting and other management systems to be designed and tested, and low fees were introduced with small but regular increases. Second, since fees were to be introduced at all levels, phasing could be carried out by cascading reforms downwards. New management systems, fees and exemptions were first implemented at large hospitals where management capacity was greatest, then cascaded downwards to lower levels. Staff at large hospitals could then use their newly acquired skills and experience to help with training and large hospitals could become the training centres for the next phase of implementation (Collins et al. 1996). Third, attention to public and staff information improved implementation prospects.

6.2 Protecting the poor while generating revenue

A major capacity failure was the design and implementation of exemption systems. This weakness was probably greatest in Ghana where incentives to charge were strongest and incentives to exempt weakest, and there were no obvious solutions as targeting according to income level is extremely difficult in practice, particularly where information is so scarce. An alternative is to abandon targeting by income level and use simpler categories for exemption which require less information, for example; age (such as under-fives), pregnant women, chronic illness sufferers (Gilson et al. 1995; Sen 1992). Another option might be to shift screening procedures away from the facility to the community where those needing exemption could be more easily identified using simple criteria (chronically ill, elderly). Community-based screening is, however, vulnerable to local patronage and abuse, and may require innovative and participatory strategies.

Another possible reform path is health insurance. Thailand had already moved along this path with a variety of insurance arrangements which generated substantial revenue for government hospitals. In Kenya, cost recovery levels improved considerably after efforts were made to tap resources from existing formal insurance schemes. Debates in Sri Lanka also focused on the potential revenue which government hospitals could tap from existing private and government health insurance schemes. In Ghana, concerns about affordability helped drive research and policy in the direction of risk sharing mechanisms and options were being evaluated for both compulsory insurance for the employed and rural community-based schemes. Nevertheless, the capacity demands that these insurance schemes are likely to place on the case study governments are probably as great as those of means tested exemptions, and they may only be a policy option in the longer term.

6.3 Capacity development

The MOH organisation and its staff do not operate in a vacuum, and their ability to perform service provision roles may be constrained by broader policy environments (Batley 1997; Grindle and Hildebrand 1995). Capacity development efforts must therefore focus on both improving systems and skills and addressing wider institutional constraints.

Existing capacity weaknesses require strengthening before new or more radical tasks, and related capacities, are developed. For example, in Ghana and Zimbabwe where routine billing, collection and accounting systems were weak, basic improvements were necessary before newer management-oriented systems could be developed.

A related question concerns the role of donors in capacity development. In Kenya, because modification of the Treasury's accounting and financial systems could not be achieved rapidly, the KHCF Project introduced a parallel reporting system which provided higher level managers with monthly revenue and expenditure data and summary reports that allowed comparison of user fee policy performance across facilities. This allowed identification of those facilities which needed supervision or audit, which in turn motivated facility managers to improve their management and reporting of cost sharing (Collins et al. 1996).

The new reporting and auditing system was a 'complementary' one however, introduced by donors (as was the case with a new financial information system in Zimbabwe: see Box 4.1, Chapter 4), so it may not be taken seriously by staff or adopted for long if an established Treasury accounting system to which all staff must adhere remains in place. This again raises the problem of tackling systems and skills within an organisation without tackling government-wide financial and accounting regulations. Referring back to Figure 5.2, the success of donor-driven capacity-building projects that attempt to develop new systems within Ministries of Health is likely to be limited if staff motivation to use these systems or learn new skills is lacking due to broader institutional factors. The problem for the donor and ministry staff at the centre is how to reward the agents it is trying to motivate and sanction poor performance, while still operating within old bureaucratic frameworks and civil service regulations.

Finally, capacity development is likely to be iterative. User fees in themselves increased local managers' financial responsibilities in Ghana and Thailand and thereby may gradually stimulate improved management skills and systems. Revenue retention in Zimbabwe should allow managers to develop financial management skills through experience, coupled with complementary training. This will help contribute to a new management culture that could provide a sound basis for future reforms – such as contracting out and increased hospital autonomy – that demand greater skills and expertise.

6
Government Purchase of Private Services

1. Introduction

This chapter explains the rationale for contractual agreements with the private sector to provide both clinical and non-clinical health services, and the expected benefits. Evidence from the four country case studies and from Thailand is used to analyse the extent to which this policy has been adopted, the forms the policy has taken and the likely problems associated with this reform measure. Particular attention is paid to the demands the policy makes on government capacity. The chapter draws conclusions on the factors constraining the more widespread adoption of contracting out, and speculates on its relevance in different country contexts.

Contractual relationships have been perceived to be central to the NPM philosophy, in two ways (Mills 1997a). First, they are seen to be the way to structure management relationships, in order to ensure clear specification of requirements by funders, and monitor the performance of providers. In this sense they apply equally to purchaser-provider relationships whether these are internal to the public sector, or between a public purchaser and private provider. Second, there is a presumption within NPM philosophy that private providers, because of their differing incentive structures, are likely to be more efficient providers of services: either because they operate in a competitive environment which forces them to be efficient if they are to survive, or because of the nature of property rights in private ownership which means they experience direct benefits from greater efficiency (Bennett, McPake and Mills 1997). Contracts appear centre stage since they are the means by which services are purchased from the private sector.

This chapter addresses contracts between public purchasers and private providers. It is thus concerned with what has been termed the 'make or buy' decision (Walsh 1995: 111). It is important to note that contractual relationships are not new: services and commodities have always needed to be purchased from the private sector. As pointed out by Larbi (1998) for Ghana, the type of activities traditionally contracted out include:

- feasibility studies for new projects;
- construction and major maintenance of buildings;
- supply, installation and maintenance of capital equipment;
- supplies, especially drugs.

Governments have always had standard procedures for handling these contracts. What is new is the widening of the range of services that may be contracted out, to encompass services traditionally provided in-house.

Contracts can take a variety of forms (Mills 1997a): they can be:

- with for-profit or not-for-profit providers;
- for a large variety of different services, such as clinical services, support services such as cleaning and catering, and management functions;
- be specified to a greater or lesser degree.

Principal–agent theory can be used to explain what sort of contracts might be required in what circumstances, as well as the characteristics of contracts found in practice. This theory, as summarised in Chapter 1, is concerned with the agency relationship, which arises out of the existence of asymmetry of information between individuals involved in a transaction. It is characterised by a principal (ill-informed individual) and agent (informed individual), both of whom seek to maximise their utility. In order to achieve his goals, the principal has to devise a contract to ensure the agent does not cheat or act opportunistically. Thus the rules within the contract are vital, including monitoring processes, as is the environment within which contracting takes place including the characteristics of the markets supplying the goods and services. In general, there are trade-offs between constraining provider opportunism, keeping transactions costs at a reasonable level, and encouraging competition for contracts (Broomberg 1994). The more that contracts try to control providers and shift risk to them, the higher the transactions costs and the less the interest in bidding. At the other extreme, a loose contract based on a long term relationship is likely to reduce incentives for efficiency. However, the nature of the service in the contract, and the ease of specifying and monitoring performance, are also crucial. The greater the difficulties of specifying and monitoring performance, the greater the argument for a closer relationship of co-operation between the two parties, as opposed to an arm's length relationship.

Principal–agent theory provides the basis on which to identify key features of contract design and implementation that will affect the performance of contracts (Mills 1997b). A framework was developed for evaluating contractual arrangements found in the case-study countries. This covered:

- the current policy on contracting; the process of developing this policy; existing contractual arrangements and their rationale;
- contract design;
- the process of awarding contracts and monitoring performance, including the availability of alternative suppliers;
- contract outcomes in terms of cost and quality;
- the presence or absence of capacities required for successful contracting.

Where possible, data were obtained and analysed on the cost and quality of particular contracts through both fieldwork for this research and drawing on a related research programme (Mills 1998), which included studies of contracting with a mine hospital in Zimbabwe (McPake and Hongoro 1995), on agreements with church hospitals in Ghana and Zimbabwe (Gilson et al. 1997), on contracting out catering services in Mumbai, India (Bhatia and Mills 1997), and on contracting for cleaning services and high-technology equipment in Thailand (Tangchar-oensathien, Nitayarumphong and Khonsawatt 1997).

This chapter considers first the contracting policies in place and their rationale. It then addresses the performance of contractual arrangements in terms of contract design, contract implementation and policy outcomes. The chapter goes on to consider the demands that contracting made on government capacity, and to what extent capacity was a constraint on performance in the various countries. The chapter ends by seeking to draw some lessons on the relevance of a policy of contracting out in low- and middle-income countries.

2.   Contracting policies and their rationale

In Ghana, contractual arrangements in place were of long standing (Smithson, Asamoa-Baah and Mills 1997). The MOH contracted out the traditional areas such as construction and major maintenance, and was required to handle drugs and supplies procurement through the Ghana Supplies Commission. There was a long-standing subsidy to church health facilities, which are major providers of services in rural areas. At the time of the study, this was done within the framework of an agreement dating from 1975, under which the MOH transferred a subsidy to the umbrella church organisation sufficient to pay the salaries of the agreed staff establishment of church facilities.

Interest had been growing in the MOH in making greater use of contractual arrangements for providing services. There were a few contracts in the past for support services, but these were not thought to have worked well. The MOH's main interest was in contracting areas of activity not seen as part of the Ministry's core business, and which patients were anyway required to pay for. At the top of the MOH agenda was contracting for catering services, since a policy of charging for meals had been introduced in 1994. The MOH's prime concern was to avoid the management burden of organising services that the public sector was obviously having difficulty running, and where expenditure control was extremely difficult. An external consultant was commissioned to investigate the feasibility of contracting-out hospital support services, including catering. He concluded that the time was not yet ripe for contracting on the grounds of both a lack of a clear public policy on services such as catering, and lack of interest in the private sector in contracts (Forster 1994). However, some progress was made in formalising performance agreements with church providers: a draft memorandum of understanding stated that there would normally be two-year rolling contracts with an annual review, the staff salary subvention would be replaced by a block grant, and there would be general specification of the services to be provided and monitoring arrangements (Ministry of Health Ghana 1998).[1] The document also stated that these arrangements could apply also to private for-profit providers, though none had yet been agreed.

Zimbabwe offered a clear contrast to Ghana. As with Ghana, there were some long-standing agreements. These included subsidies to church hospitals, in particular an arrangement dating from 1969 where block grants were given to church hospitals to act as the local district hospital. As in Ghana, the agreement did not specify the services that should be provided, or cost and quality outputs. A similar arrangement had existed for a long time with a mine hospital, though paid on a fee per patient basis, to provide services to the local population (McPake and Hongoro 1995). However, Zimbabwe had greater experience of support service contracts, admittedly arranged in the past on a rather *ad hoc* basis, and also a new comprehensive policy had been put in place. The Cabinet had approved contracting out as a policy option for ministries in 1994, and the MOH was one of the first ministries to develop contracting out proposals. The key government objectives were to:

- reduce the number of civil servants and public expenditure;
- promote the local business sector;
- improve efficiency and effectiveness of public services;
- improve public management.

External support was provided to both the government and the MOH in developing options and recommendations. The MOH had decided to focus on support services and to phase in the policy, starting first with the simplest service (security) at the four central hospitals and a new provincial hospital; catering, considered to be the most complex service, was to be last. However, the MOH was instructed by the Public Service Commission to include all five services (security, grounds maintenance, cleaning, catering, laundry) in the first phase. By 1999, central hospitals contracted out most of their laundry, equipment maintenance, grounds maintenance and security. Similar arrangements were introduced at those provincial hospitals where the availability of local suppliers made this feasible.

In India, World Bank policy documents had asserted a considerable potential for the contracting out of various aspects of health services (Bennett and Muraleedharan 1998). They suggested that support services at hospitals should be contracted out 'whenever feasible', that contracting out of mainstream diagnostic services and clinical services be evaluated; that contracting out should be used in the delivery of national disease control programmes, and that NGOs be contracted to provide primary health care in some remote rural areas. Government documents had acknowledged the potential importance of contracting, but suggested a more limited role: in new areas where the public sector was not involved, and in areas where the public sector might be inefficient such as security, catering, cleaning and laundry.

In Tamil Nadu, contracting out had not been a main thrust of health sector reforms, though there were a number of small-scale, relatively recent contractual arrangements in the health sector. These included contracts for hospital equipment maintenance, for high technology diagnostic services, and for IEC campaigns by the AIDS society, and planned laundry contracting. There was some external encouragement involved in some of these: for example, the contract for hospital equipment maintenance had been encouraged by seed funding from the Government of India, and since AIDS control received substantial World Bank funding it is likely that this was a factor in encouraging contracting of advertising. In contrast, in Mumbai, there was considerable contracting out of support services in hospitals owned by the municipal corporation. The range of services contracted out included catering, laundry, housekeeping, hospital maintenance, security, waste disposal, importation procedures and residual spraying in one area (Bhatia and Mills 1997). Contracting appeared not to be a recent policy, and arrangements were of long standing.

Sri Lanka had no contracting out of clinical services, and no major plans to do so. Contracting out had happened by necessity in the past, when government laboratory technicians had gone on strike, and was being considered for bypass surgery because of long waiting lists in the central hospital. In contrast, contracting of support services was quite common: for example, at both central and provincial hospitals, laundry and security were normally contracted out, and at small hospitals, cooking was commonly done by the contractor providing food supplies.

Thailand had had quite extensive contracting of support services for some time, done at hospital initiative within strict central regulations. In recent years such regulations had begun to be relaxed in order to facilitate contracting out, including permitting contracting out in existing buildings and not just new ones. A key event marking a significant change in policy was a Cabinet resolution in 1994 on reforming the civil service and limiting its size. It proposed that the posts of janitor, cleaner and driver be gradually cut from the establishment as people retired, and envisaged that in the future all these services would be contracted out. No similar regulations existed for contracting-out of clinical services for the general public. While individual hospitals could propose arrangements to the Ministry of Finance, the process of approval was slow. Contractual arrangements had developed with respect to the contracting out of the provision and maintenance of high technology equipment, largely to secure up-to-date machines and high standards of maintenance. Though one hospital involved had been a government hospital, all others were university hospitals which had much greater autonomy and could take such decisions themselves.

However, it is important to note that contracts were the basis of service provision for the social insurance scheme introduced in 1991. Employers (and subsequently employees) chose annually a 'contractor hospital', which could be public or private, to provide their health care. Such hospitals were then contracted by the social security office.

From this review of contracting out policy, some clear differences can be seen between the countries. Zimbabwe appeared the most advanced in terms of pursuing an NPM rationale for contracting out and adopting a formal policy, and had had external support and encouragement to do so. Thailand appeared to be on a similar track, but was purely internally driven. Ghana had aspirations to such a policy, but was at the very early stages of working out feasibility, and it was not very clear whether the interest in contracting was locally generated or externally influenced. In India and Sri Lanka, NPM arguments for contracting out were not prominent. External encouragement, although present, had not led to any major shift in policy.

However, the degree of prominence of NPM arguments did not match the actual extent of contracting out. Those countries where NPM arguments were least prominent in fact had the greatest number of arrangements, though it is important to note that most common was the contracting out of support services, and least common the contracting out of clinical services, and that contracted services were not numerous and accounted for a very small proportion of the government health budget. Contracting to NGOs, including church organisations, existed implicitly, in the sense that subsidies were provided, but with little written specification of services to be provided. These implicit arrangements were particularly common in the two African countries, but also existed elsewhere.

The following section considers the performance of contracting-out arrangements including issues and problems in contract design, issues in the process of implementation, and the policy outcomes. The choice of arrangements to study was limited by the arrangements in existence; those included were:

- Ghana: contracts with church organisations (drawing from Gilson et al. 1997);
- Zimbabwe: the early phases of implementing the new contracting out policy for support services; contracts with church organisations (drawing from Gilson et al. 1997) and the contract for district hospital services with a mine hospital (drawing from McPake and Hongoro 1995);
- India: contracting for laundry services, high-technology equipment, equipment maintenance services and advertising for AIDS control in Tamil Nadu; catering contracts in Mumbai (drawing from Bhatia and Mills 1997);
- Sri Lanka: food procurement;
- Thailand: contracting for high technology equipment and cleaning (drawing from Tancharoensathien, Nitayarumphong and Khonsawatt 1997).

3.   Contract performance

3.1   Contract design

Aspects of contract design that are key to both the nature of contracts and their likely performance are the specification of the service; the pricing method; the duration of the contract; and specification of sanctions for poor performance (Mills 1998).

Service specification

Service specification appeared generally more straightforward for support services than for clinical services. For example, the MOH in Zimbabwe had been able to draw up such contracts:

> This was easier to do for things like security and grounds maintenance. With laundry and catering we are still facing problems.... but the UK experience and the assistance we have received from the PSC [Public Service Comission], ODA [Overseas Development Administration] and other consultants is allowing us to design these contracts also. (Russell et al. 1997).

Other countries also seemed to face few difficulties in specifying such contracts. In Chennai and Mumbai there were standard contracts that were used. The key difficulty was when quality standards were needed, as in the case of catering. Catering contracts in Mumbai, for example, were criticised for their lack of quality standards for cooked meals (Bhatia and Mills 1997). In contrast, in Sri Lanka where most arrangements involved the supply of raw produce, although quality standards were vague this had not been perceived as a problem because poor quality produce could readily be identified (e.g. rotten vegetables).

In Ghana, service specification seemed a greater difficulty. It was said, for example, that there were frequently problems with specification of contracts let through central tender board procedures: for example, in the past there had been food contracts which had specified neither quantities nor price. Poor wording of terms of reference was also said to be a problem in contracting for private management services.

The only examples of contracts for clinical services were those for high-technology services in India and Thailand, the mine hospital in Zimbabwe, insured workers in Thailand, and contracts with NGOs. The first type had presented few service specification problems in technical terms, perhaps the reason for the popularity of contractual arrangements for such services. However the arrangements differed between the two countries: in Tamil Nadu the arrangement was largely the creation of a commercial service within a public hospital: the hospital provided space without charge, but otherwise all resources were paid and managed by the contractor, including clinical staff. In contrast, in Thailand the clinical input came from the hospital, thus ensuring greater control over service provision.

In the social insurance arrangements in Thailand, specification concerned the type of hospital eligible to be a main contractor, and the nature of services to be provided by the contractor. The former consisted primarily of specification of service infrastructure such as number of beds, range of specialities, levels of equipment and provision of information on treatments provided to insured workers. The specification of services to be provided simply stated that the contractor would provide services to all outpatient and inpatient cases within the capitation rate[2], and that services would be provided until the insured person had regained his or her full health (Bennett et al. 1998). While there was concern that not all contractor hospitals had been meeting this specification, reform proposals had concentrated on improving information provision, monitoring procedures and introducing an accreditation system rather than on tightening up the specification of services to be provided.

In Ghana and Zimbabwe, agreements with NGOs were simply not specified, presumably because the MOH counted on goodwill and common interest being sufficient motivation. However, in both countries there was discussion of moving to a more explicit contract, with concrete progress being made in Ghana, as stated earlier.

A key feature of most contracts was that they were arranged for new services, and involved no staff redundancies. This was the case with catering services in Mumbai, for example. The difficulties in India of contracting out existing services was shown by the experience of Tamil Nadu: the Department of Health had attempted to contract out laundry services in a hospital, but found that it could not lay off existing staff; the contractor was not willing to employ them; and the staff were not willing to be employed by the contractor. After a year of negotiation, the government had abandoned the plan to contract. In contrast, in Zimbabwe the MOH was successful in implementing the first phase of its contracting plans which involved contracting out existing services[3], even though during elections the contracting out policy was temporarily abandoned by the Cabinet to avoid potential conflict with government workers. Measures were taken to help staff who would lose their jobs to set up companies to bid for contracts, with over 200 such companies being created (personal communication, Director Public Services Commission) and private companies were told they had a better chance of winning contracts if they offered to absorb some of the existing workforce.

Pricing methods

For support services, both Thailand and Mumbai had arrangements whereby the price was set in advance, and firms asked to bid what service they would provide for that price. This took the form of a price per meal in the two contracts in Mumbai, and a price per square metre in cleaning contracts in Thailand. Such arrangements have the advantage of making the total cost of the contract more predictable; however, there is a danger of keeping the price too low and discouraging bids (this seemed to be the case in both arrangements). There was an interesting difference in Sri Lanka between pricing arrangements for private suppliers selected through competition and for a cooperative selected without competition to supply food to one hospital. The prices for the latter were adjusted monthly if necessary, whereas for the former they were fixed for a year. Given the fluctuation of food prices over the year, suppliers with a fixed annual price could face difficulties in supplying food within their price ceiling, and felt that as a result food quality could suffer.

The desirability of different pricing methods for clinical services is hotly debated in the literature (Barnum, Saxenian and Kutzin 1995), especially the relative merits and dangers of fee-for-service, case-based and capitation payment. The two high technology examples, from Thailand and Tamil Nadu, involved user fees which were paid via the hospital (in the former) and direct to the contractor (in the latter). Given the nature of the technology, there are few concerns about excessive use of these services unless there were informal payments to staff to encourage them to make excessive numbers of referrals. The payment arrangement for the mine hospital in Zimbabwe also involved fee for service – per inpatient day and per outpatient. Although only those who could not pay should have received free treatment, in practice the screening of patients was ineffective and the hospital had no incentive to ensure that those who should pay, did so. As a result, the cost of the contract was higher than it should have been and absorbed an excessive share of total provincial expenditure. The social insurance scheme in Thailand used capitation payment and as a result, costs had been very successfully contained (Tancharoensathein, Nitayarumphong and Khonsawatt 1999), and the administrative demands of the payment system minimised. However concerns had emerged that private hospitals had restricted service provision in order to increase their profits (Mills et al. 1999). It is clear that no payment method for clinical services is without potential problems, and that each method involves the possibility that unscrupulous contractors may exploit the payment method in their own interest.

Contract duration

Support service contracts were commonly for one year. Staff of the MOH in Zimbabwe, however, felt that longer contracts might be preferable in the first instance in order to stimulate bids and encourage firms to invest in service development and the specific expertise required for hospital services, and to provide time for both sides to develop skills and mutual understanding, and resolve problems.

Contracts (or agreements) for clinical services were often of unspecified duration, reflecting their rather different nature. Even where a duration was specified (e.g. high technology equipment in Thailand) this was very long.

Sanctions for poor performance

Poor contract specification means inevitably that sanctions for poor performance will be limited, even if there is specific provision in contracts for sanctions. For example, catering contracts in Mumbai had made provision for fines for poor performance, but since quality standards were not clearly stated in the contract, it would have been difficult to impose them. Similarly with the mine hospital agreement, although there was provision for termination of the contract with three months' notice on either side, there was no formal process for monitoring the quality of services or the operation of the contract at the time of the study (McPake and Hongoro 1993).

3.2   Contract implementation

Key issues and problems encountered in implementing contractual arrangements were the degree of competition, transparency in the process of awarding contracts, and allocation of responsibilities for agreeing and monitoring contractor performance.

Degree of competition

Table 6.1 summarises the arrangements for agreeing contracts, and in particular whether or not they were competitively awarded. In general it seems that support service contracts were commonly awarded competitively, with one exception in Sri Lanka where non-competitive arrangements of the 1960s and 1970s involving raw food supply by government sponsored non-profit bodies such as co-operatives still persisted at some smaller hospitals.

Table 6.1 Process of awarding contracts

Country	Support service contracts	Clinical contracts
Ghana	*	Agreements with church organisations: • negotiated
Zimbabwe	Contracts not yet awarded at time of study; to be awarded competitively; competition expected to be limited outside Harare	Agreements with church organisations and mining hospital: • negotiated • no alternative suppliers in short term
India	Catering in Mumbai hospitals: • awarded competitively • large number of potential suppliers • few bids • change of contractor rare Equipment maintenance: • negotiated • would require multiple contracts if alternative suppliers used, since only the current supplier could maintain all types of equipment	High technology equipment: • negotiated despite many potential suppliers AIDS control adverts: • competitive • many bidders
Sri Lanka	Provision of hospital food: • three awarded competitively; few bidders • one negotiated with Coop	*
Thailand	Cleaning services: • awarded competitively • large number of potential suppliers • reasonable number of bids, though not from high quality firms	High technology equipment: • usually negotiated despite many potential suppliers • contractor dominated terms of contract Social insurance scheme: • insured worker annually selected health service provider from approved list of hospitals (both public and private)

* None studied.

In contrast, contracts for clinical services were not awarded competitively except in Thailand, for some of the contracts for high technology equipment and for health care provision for workers insured under the social insurance scheme, who could annually select their health service provider.

It is noteworthy that even with the support service contracts, the degree of actual competition was often very limited. This was perhaps most obvious in Mumbai, where problems of availability of suppliers for catering contracts might not have been expected. In Mumbai and also Thailand, one reason for the small number of bidders may have been the practice of fixing the price in the tender, which probably made the contract unattractive to many potential suppliers. Certainly the cleaning price for Bangkok was well below what firms could have earned at that time from private sector contracts. Another reason, suggested by the case study in Sri Lanka, is that suppliers had created a cartel. Anecdotal evidence suggested that suppliers organised and decided who would win a particular contract, and might even create an appearance of competition by ensuring some bids were submitted with inflated prices. This may also have been the case in Mumbai, and is a recognised problem more generally in India. An alternative or additional explanation may be that the award of contracts was known to be biased to a particular supplier; hence it was not worth the effort for other firms to bid.

Transparency

Firm information on the process of awarding contracts was hard to obtain. However, there was concern in several of the countries that the process was not transparent, and might be influenced by those who stood to gain. In Ghana, Larbi (1998) commented that in the teaching hospitals and other decentralised units, contracting out decisions were sometimes monopolised by a few powerful individuals, which could lead to charges that contracts were used as avenues for rent-seeking and patronage. In Thailand, there had been a succession of scandals about illegal payments to politicians in major contracts and purchasing decisions (Bennett et al. 1998).

Allocation of responsibilities for contract implementation and monitoring

Health service contracts normally involve a service provided at a local unit; hence a key issue is the extent of involvement of that unit (usually a hospital) in the contracting process. In Zimbabwe, for each hospital and each service to be contracted out, the tender board was to include hospital staff with relevant expertise. In Mumbai and Thailand, the contracting process also seemed to involve hospital staff fully. In Ghana, however, tender board procedures were criticised as having very little involvement of MOH staff. For example, a cleaning contract had given rise to problems because the contract was agreed centrally and the hospital had had little say.

In general, contract monitoring was seen as a problem, whether because contract specification was weak, making monitoring difficult; or information on which to monitor was lacking; or staff lacked the motivation to monitor; or it was not made clear whose responsibility it was to monitor. For example, it was seen as a problem in the Sri Lanka study that the delegation of responsibility and authority to hospitals to monitor the contract and take punitive action was not clear: formal authority was vested with the province.

3.3   Policy outcomes

Where possible, either quantitative or qualitative information was sought on the relative cost and quality of the contracted service as compared to the service when directly provided, and on managers' views on contract performance. The results are summarised in Table 6.2. The Thai social insurance contracts were omitted since there was no obvious alternative arrangement for comparison.

A large number of different factors are likely to explain these results. There is some evidence that in India, Sri Lanka and Thailand private contractors were capable of supplying support services such as food and cleaning at a cost to the public sector that was lower than if the government had provided those services itself. However, there was also evidence that the lower cost was achieved at the expense of quality: for example, lower quality meals in Mumbai hospitals. In this case, however, the margin between the cost of the contracted service and direct provision was so great that a higher price could have been paid for the contract to obtain higher quality, while still generating savings. The main reason for greater private sector efficiency is likely to have been lower labour costs. Whether this reflected greater productivity, and/or lower wages, varied between the countries.

In Sri Lanka, there had also appeared to be a cost quality trade-off, with a danger that quality might be driven down to unacceptable levels. The study permitted a comparison between competitively awarded contracts and one that was negotiated, and between private, for-profit suppliers and co-operatives. There was no evidence of poorer performance of the latter. Indeed, one district medical officer commented: 'it does not matter if the food supplier is a cooperative or private, it is strict supervision that is required' (Russell and Attanayake 1997).

Table 6.2 Evidence on policy outcomes: comparison of contracted-out service with directly provided government service

	Support service contracts	Clinical contracts
Ghana	*	Agreements with church organisations: • *Cost:* similar • *Quality:* largely similar • *Managers' comments*: church hospitals had advantages of greater staff commitment and more autonomy in resource use decisions
Zimbabwe	**	Agreement with church organisations: • *Cost:* lower • *Quality:* largely similar • *Managers' comments*: church hospitals had advantages of greater staff commitment and more autonomy Agreement with mine hospital: • *Cost:* contractor price for inpatients lower than government; for outpatients higher • *Quality:* at least as good • *Managers' comments*: little attention paid to contract
India	Catering contracts in Mumbai hospitals: • *Cost:* lower • *Quality:* lower • *Managers' comments*: contracting had advantages e.g. reduced administrative burden Equipment maintenance: • *Cost:* no data • *Quality:* managers complained of slow response time • *Managers' comments*: contract expensive but no convenient alternative	High technology equipment contracts: • *Cost:* borne by users; much cheaper than private services • *Quality:* longer opening hours; functioning equipment; staff dissatisfied with pay • *Managers' comments*: private sector better able to secure higher staff productivity

133

Table 6.2 (*continued*)

	Support service contracts	Clinical contracts
Sri Lanka	Competitive contracts for provision of hospital food:*** • *Cost*: negotiated contract more costly • *Quality*: lower food quality with competitive contracts • *Managers' comments*: cost minimisation is main aim; achieved by competition	*
Thailand	Cleaning service contracts: • *Cost*: probably slightly lower • *Quality*: probably better • *Managers' comments*: more satisfied with contracted service	High technology equipment contracts: • *Cost*: varying pattern: some cheaper, others more expensive • *Quality*: better maintenance and productivity • *Managers' comments*: advantages of higher productivity and improved access

* None studied.
** No evidence.
*** Comparison was between competitively awarded contracts and directly negotiated contract.
Note: 'Cost' represents the cost to the government of contracting-out (not the cost to the contractor of providing the service); 'managers' are those at hospital level.

Indeed, the willingness of hospital staff to supervise contractor performance seemed key in several of the studies. The Mumbai evaluation had indicated that this was a problem, though also pointed out that supervision was made more difficult by the lack of performance standards specified in the contract.

A further explanation for these findings is the pricing arrangements. In Mumbai, those arrangements with low cost and low quality were where the hospital had set the price in the tender. Similarly in Sri Lanka, a major explanation for poor quality food was not the contractual arrangements *per se*, but rather the pricing arrangement where the price was set for the whole year in a situation where food prices could vary markedly from month to month.

Managers' views provided information which was complementary to that obtained on costs and quality, and also shed light on reasons for differences in performance of directly provided and contracted out services. Managers consistently preferred contracting out arrangements for support services, arguing that they removed from them the difficulties of managing services which involved problems of staff relations and control of supplies. In India and Sri Lanka, a further advantage was the protection that contracting out provided from public sector strikes and industrial relations problems with unskilled labour categories.

The essence of the arrangements for clinical services, with the exception of the social insurance arrangement in Thailand, was that they had made services available which the state was not in a position to provide or which it did not make sense for the state to duplicate. This was the case, for example, with the church hospitals in Ghana and Zimbabwe, and the mine hospital in Zimbabwe. Thus the specific terms of the agreement were not the key consideration for decision makers, and an orientation towards specifying and monitoring performance was not part of the government management culture. The fact that church facilities were believed to function in the interests of the general population was a further reason for both funding them and not having close monitoring arrangements. Where facilities such as those run by the churches were believed to function better than similar government services, a consistent explanation was the greater degree of autonomy they enjoyed, which enabled better management. Church facilities were also believed to benefit from greater staff motivation, which meant they obtained higher performance at no extra cost.

In the case of contracts for high-technology services, those in Thailand had performed better than direct provision, no doubt due to the direct financial interest of the operators in ensuring functioning machines (since otherwise the machines would not generate income). In Chennai, lack of access to capital had meant that direct provision was not an option, though again the contractor's dependence on fee revenue provided an incentive to minimise downtime.

4.   The demands on government capacity

The preceding sections, in exploring the problems associated with contracting and seeking to explain performance, at various points referred to issues that relate to government capacity to design, implement and monitor contracts. This section seeks to bring these issues together, and to examine to what extent capacity was indeed a constraint on performance in the various countries. The section first examines capacity to contract taking countries in pairs on the basis of presenting similar capacity problems, and then seeks to draw some general lessons.

4.1   Ghana and Zimbabwe

There was clear evidence in Ghana that lack of skills and experience amongst MOH staff was a key constraint in making progress with support service contracting, as well as an important explanation for slow progress with performance agreements with church facilities. Senior staff had found it difficult to formulate a policy because of both limitations of expertise and lack of time to devote to this one issue.[4] Attempts were made to relax this constraint by using an external consultant who could draw on UK experience, but the result was not considered very helpful, partly because the model considered desirable was one where both the existing service providers and private providers would be encouraged to bid in competition with each other. This implied organising the in-house service on a commercial basis, which was not considered feasible in the short term. In contrast, Zimbabwe did find UK experience helpful: while one explanation may be a more suitable choice of consultant in the case of Zimbabwe, it is also likely to be the case that external advice is most helpful when there is expertise within the country to brief consultants and interpret advice. Zimbabwe appeared to have a more skilled group of managers in the MOH, who in addition were provided both with training and with study tours to learn about UK experience.

Information availability and use was another key problem. Both countries had a very poor knowledge of their own costs, and information systems from which service costs could not readily be extracted. This made it difficult for the MOH to judge when contracting might be an efficient option and to evaluate bids. Both countries were receiving support to reform financial information systems, but this would take time before costing information became more routinely available. It was recognised that information availability was not sufficient if staff were poorly motivated to maintain information systems or act on the information. Both countries had experienced problems in paying on time: potential private sector suppliers perceived this to be an important deterrent to bidding for government contracts. In Zimbabwe, the process of contracting out had been aided by reforms which allowed hospitals at all levels to keep revenue in a fund which could be easily accessed by hospital managers.

In both Ghana and Zimbabwe, it was anticipated that attempts to contract out existing services would encounter strong union and worker opposition. In Ghana, this was yet a further reason for slow progress, but interestingly was overcome in Zimbabwe. One reason is likely to be the fact that the contracting out policy was adopted at a high level (by Cabinet) and hence the MOH had clear backing for its plans. This did not appear to be the case in Ghana. Another reason was likely to have been the attention paid in Zimbabwe to arrangements for affected workers. They were encouraged to set up their own companies to bid for contracts, and firms winning contracts were asked to take on former hospital employees for a trial period of a year, after which they could be dismissed if their performance was poor. This had also helped ensure that the knowledge and expertise of affected hospital employees were not totally lost.

A further contrast is provided by differing levels of private sector capacity. In Ghana, it seemed that private sector capacity to take on government contracts for support services was very limited, even in Accra (Forster 1994). Moreover, private sector wages were higher, so any efficiency advantages of a private sector supplier would have to come solely from higher productivity and better management of resources. The private sector in Zimbabwe was more developed, especially in Harare, and there seemed to be less concern that private costs might be higher. In addition, MOH managers had thought through strategies for encouraging private sector participation in what might be regarded as a risky venture: for example offering longer term contracts, and seeking to work with contractors to overcome teething problems. Support services do not always require substantial initial investment (e.g. cleaning; security), and other services can be organised in such as way as to minimise such requirements (e.g. rental of hospital-owned cooking and laundry equipment). Hence access to capital does not need to be a major constraint on private sector participation and other factors (ability to organise; level of trust in government as a payer; availability of more profitable business opportunities) are likely to be more powerful in explaining the level of capacity and degree of interest of the private sector.

Neither government had given much consideration to contracting for clinical services with for-profit providers. It was briefly mentioned in Ghanaian policy documents as a strategy for provision of primary care services in under-served areas, though these tended not to be areas where the for-profit formal private sector was very active. Zimbabwe had a substantial formal private sector, but contractual relationships with such providers did not appear to be on the agenda, probably because they were located in urban areas where the government already had its own services, and possibly because they were known or believed to be expensive. The experience of the contract with the mine hospital had not been a positive one, and had highlighted capacity weaknesses in the MOH and provincial level to design and monitor such contracts (McPake and Hongoro 1995). It is likely that both governments were more comfortable engaging in agreements with non profit providers, and more doubtful of the motivations of for-profit providers and of government ability to ensure ethical behaviour.

4.2 India and Sri Lanka

India and Sri Lanka shared a system of administration that functioned reasonably well, if in a centralised and bureaucratic way. In general, skills were present to design and negotiate contracts for support services, though not at all levels in Sri Lanka, and standard contract forms were available. Although the governments did not always pay on time, they did pay eventually. However, government systems did not operate in a very flexible fashion – witness the fixed price approach which had clear deficiencies. Also staff motivation to supervise and monitor contracts was consistently identified as a problem.

Constraints to the greater use of contracting were more political than administrative. In both countries a clear constraint was the inability to retrench public sector workers and to address the power of the public service unions in dictating employment terms and conditions. In Sri Lanka, public and trade union opposition to 'privatisation' had rendered politicians reluctant to take any action that might be construed as such, and contracting-out was simply not on the agenda of the MOH:

> If we sent any proposals to Cabinet to introduce fees, or to contract out medical services to private suppliers, they would simply be thrown out. They would have strikes and even riots on their hands. (Russell and Attanayake 1997)

In both countries, private sector capacity existed to take on contracts for most support services, although there were concerns that markets were not very competitive, either because of action by suppliers to limit competition, or because government prices and procedures discouraged substantial numbers of bidders.

4.3   Thailand

Thailand also had the capacities to handle contracting. However, government procedures were still very centralised and bureaucratic, and the Thai government had some way to go to adapt its systems to create a more flexible approach to service provision. It was also not taking advantages of the opportunities the private sector presented to encourage competition for contracts, and to exercise government purchasing power to obtain favourable terms.

Thailand is the one country, of those studied, which had had extensive experience of contracting with for-profit health care providers. This experience, in the context of a capitation payment system in the contracts, highlighted the importance in clinical contracting of not relying solely on written agreements, but rather on creating broader systems of monitoring and accountability (Mills et al. 1999). For example, the media, which in Thailand was quite active, had played an important role in publicising cases where private hospitals had under provided services to the insured, and had helped to raise awareness of their rights amongst those insured. Other institutional developments were also necessary: for example, an active Medical Council to ensure high standards of professional ethics.

4.4   General overview

Looking overall at all study countries, while capacity within the MOH was important in managing the detail of contracts, it appeared that either this capacity was there, or could be built up with some effort and commitment and external support. More important and fundamental constraints to a greater use of contracting were external to the MOH. These included unreformed and centralised bureaucratic systems that provided little flexibility in how contracts were specified and managed and that gave managers little authority or responsibility; inability to address the labour implications of contracting; and lack of political backing to pursue courses of action unpopular with public sector workers. Health services are labour-intensive, and hence managing the labour implications of reform is a central concern. It is perhaps relevant that the substantial extension of contracting for support services in the UK occurred at a time when legislation was weakening the power of organised labour, and also that support services employed low-skilled workers with limited influence. In contrast, in developing countries public sector workers generally are in a more privileged position, and in the study countries had some considerable power, especially in India and Sri Lanka, to impede change.

Although the issue was not very explicit in the country case studies, a frequent concern of managers encouraged to expand contractual arrangements is the scope this provides for corruption. In Sri Lanka and Thailand, for example, government contracting procedures were known to be influenced by bribes promised to politicians (Russell and Attenayake 1998, Bennett et al. 1998), and corruption in contracting procedures has been noted in other countries (Lalta 1993, Berachochea 1997).

Indeed, the NPM concept of contracting involves an important shift from service provision based on bureaucratic hierarchies to market-based provision involving competitive bidding, contract allocation and management, and quality and cost control at arms length. These imply very different sorts of relationships between the various parties (Flynn 1999): competitive bidding requires firms that do not coordinate with each other over the bidding process; there should be no exchange of gifts in the bidding process between governments and providers; monitoring of contractors needs to be based on the contracts backed by law. Although contracts may be designed and implemented, this does not mean that the conditions for the contracting process to operate as intended actually exist. While this research was not able to explore in depth the nature of the contractual and market relationships, there were certainly grounds for believing that relationships between government and contractors were often not at arm's length and transparent, and that markets were not fully competitive. It is likely that changes towards market-based relationships will be protracted, and that building up technical competence to handle contracts is only part of what is needed.

5.   Conclusions

Figure 6.1 summarises the influences on contracting policy drawn out in this chapter, and highlights the reasons for the lack of more widespread adoption of a policy of contracting out.

Of the core countries, only Zimbabwe had appeared to be seeking to implement a policy of contracting out based on NPM principles. Evidence from elsewhere suggests that this conclusion is not atypical of low-income countries in general: there is more discussion than actual action (Mills and

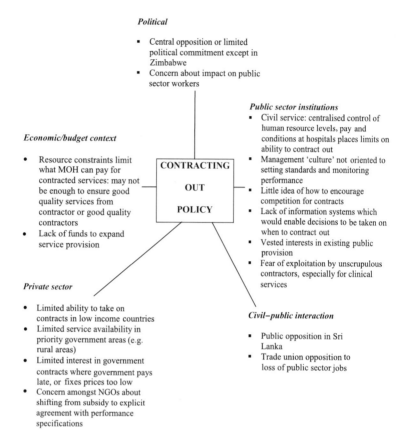

Political

- Central opposition or limited political commitment except in Zimbabwe
- Concern about impact on public sector workers

Economic/budget context

- Resource constraints limit what MOH can pay for contracted services: may not be enough to ensure good quality services from contractor or good quality contractors
- Lack of funds to expand service provision

CONTRACTING OUT POLICY

Public sector institutions

- Civil service: centralised control of human resource levels, pay and conditions at hospitals places limits on ability to contract out
- Management 'culture' not oriented to setting standards and monitoring performance
- Little idea of how to encourage competition for contracts
- Lack of information systems which would enable decisions to be taken on when to contract out
- Vested interests in existing public provision
- Fear of exploitation by unscrupulous contractors, especially for clinical services

Private sector

- Limited ability to take on contracts in low income countries
- Limited service availability in priority government areas (e.g. rural areas)
- Limited interest in government contracts where government pays late, or fixes prices too low
- Concern amongst NGOs about shifting from subsidy to explicit agreement with performance specifications

Civil–public interaction

- Public opposition in Sri Lanka
- Trade union opposition to loss of public sector jobs

Figure 6.1 Influences on contracting out policy: the political, institutional and economic constraints

Broomberg 1998). Thailand also was moving in that direction, but in an economic environment which offered much greater scope for contracting out. Some forms of contractual relationships did exist in all the countries, but the motivations for setting them up were quite diverse, and in general did not derive from a NPM agenda. Although these arrangements were studied, this was done to provide insights into the problems associated with contracting out and the necessary government capacities required, rather than as an evaluation of NPM *per se*. The key reasons identified in Figure 6.1 for the very limited adoption of contracting out as a policy include lack of political support; a variety of factors associated with public sector institutions; and lack of capacity or interest in the private sector.

The introduction to this chapter identified two rationales for contracting within the NPM approach: to structure management relationships, and to benefit from the greater efficiency of private suppliers. There was awareness of both these rationales amongst governments, but some scepticism over whether the private sector was necessarily more efficient, and whether the contracting process could really ensure that the contractor performed according to the contract and did not exploit the contract. This caused greater concern with respect to clinical services than support services. The awareness of the value of explicit arrangements was most evident in relation to agreements with church providers in the two African countries, though the church providers themselves were concerned about the introduction of performance agreements in a relationship which they felt should be based on mutual trust (Gilson et al. 1997). The fact that large numbers of public sector workers would be affected by any widespread policy of contracting out and would thus oppose it was a powerful explanation for the lack of a policy on support service contracting in India and Sri Lanka. Greater contracting out of clinical services was not an obvious strategy where governments already had an extensive network of services, and, even where services were inadequate, this policy was constrained by lack of funds to extend services and the fact that areas with few public services were also those with few private providers.

Arrangements in countries appeared to suggest that formal contractual arrangements were most appropriate for hospital support services and some management functions. Formal and competitively awarded clinical contracts were quite rare, not just because of the historical dominance of the state in the formal medical sector as reviewed in Chapter 3, but also because of the nature of the services provided. It was clear, as implied by principal–agent theory, that formal contracts were developed for services that were easier to specify, and that less formal, trust-based arrangements were more common for clinical services where performance was less easy to specify or monitor and the user was in weak position to exercise informed choice or check on performance.

For services where contracting was appropriate, how severe a constraint was capacity? For support services, government capacity was a clear constraint only in Ghana and to a slightly lesser extent in Zimbabwe; for clinical services, since few arrangements were in place, it was not possible to draw firm conclusions though clinical contracts do make greater demands on capacity. Key missing elements in internal capacity were the ability to make judgements on contracting out based on knowledge of the costs of direct service provision, and skills such as those required for contract design, negotiation and monitoring which are acquired through experience (Bennett and Mills 1998).

Capacity constraints external to the MOH were even more important; in particular the rules and regulations relating to public sector workers, public sector tendering procedures which made it difficult to involve the right levels of managers in contract design and monitoring, and financial systems which could not guarantee timely payment.

Finally, the level of development of the private sector was a severe constraint in the low -income countries, especially outside the capital city, making it difficult to ensure competition for contracts and suggesting that in such circumstances, negotiation with a trustworthy supplier may be better tactic if services need to be obtained from outside the MOH.

This analysis suggests that in terms of the relevance of a contracting out policy, three different categories of country can be distinguished.

1. Countries with both very limited government capacity to know how to go about contracting and limited private sector capacity to contract (e.g. Ghana). Here, it is unlikely to be feasible to use contracting on an extensive basis, though it might be used in the capital city for some support services, and in the form of performance agreements for services provided by NGOs and church organisations.
2. Countries with competent administrations and fairly extensive private sectors but limited interest in government contracts because of low prices and/or late payment (e.g. Sri Lanka, India). Measures are needed to improve government handling of contracts, and to encourage competition and interest in contracts. However, in Sri Lanka and India at least, more widespread use of contracts is dependent on a fundamental change in the attitudes of politicians and civil servants, and relaxation of regulations relating to public sector worker employment.
3. Countries with competent administrations and extensive private sectors with a high level of competition (e.g. Thailand). Measures needed here are those which will encourage competition and remove regulations that inhibit competition for government contracts.

In all countries, competitive contractual arrangements are more readily applied to support services than clinical services, and the latter are likely to require a particularly supportive environment to work well.

7
Regulating and Enabling the Private Sector

1. Background to policy change

New Public Management protagonists argue that the private sector can play an important role in service delivery. A variety of theoretical arguments have been used to support such an approach. For example, some economic theorists argue that few health services have characteristics which mean that they cannot be provided by the market. Indeed, for most personal, curative, health services, markets are likely to exist; however, they are likely to function imperfectly due to problems of asymmetric information.

New Institutional Economics also provides arguments supporting the importance of a vibrant private sector. Government provision of services is commonly monopolistic, hence, it is argued, there are few incentives for efficient behaviour, high quality care or responsiveness to consumers amongst public health providers. If private sector provision is promoted, then by ensuring that there are alternative sources of health care this gives people greater opportunity to vote with their feet. Furthermore, in contrast to public sector providers, private providers (due to their profit motive) have a very direct incentive to be responsive to consumers and maintain efficient services. This set of arguments has been used not only in the health sector but throughout many other sectors of the economy (Roth 1988).

A variety of pragmatic arguments have also been made to support private sector development in health care. For example, a key World Bank paper suggested that private sector development may expand access, reduce the administrative and financial burdens upon government, and possibly increase overall sectoral efficiency (World Bank 1987).

These arguments in favour of expanding private sector development do not ignore the likely problems which private sector expansion might bring. For example, analysts often note the significant informational failures within the health sector for services (such as curative personal care) which are otherwise much like many goods normally traded in the market. The proposed solution to such market failure is expansion of the government role in information provision (Musgrove 1996). Problems associated with a tendency amongst private for-profit providers to underprovide services they cannot readily charge for, or to focus on those aspects of care which consumers may readily measure, or to concentrate in urban areas, have all been noted. Effective health sector regulation is seen as the key to resolving these problems (World Bank 1993), however concrete proposals on how best to strengthen regulation are largely absent.

The possible reasons for promoting the private sector (as discussed above) are diverse. Accordingly, the measures which government have adopted in this reform area are also diverse: some are explicitly targeted at expanding private sector provision; some are targeted at regulating (generally to improve quality of) existing private sector provision; and some measures (such as social health insurance development) are pursued for an entirely separate purpose but can have far-reaching and often unanticipated effects upon the private sector. Table 7.1 categorises broadly the types of measures governments have taken in this area.

These measures may be targeted at all private providers, but it is common for interventions to distinguish between (i) non-profit and for-profit private providers and (ii) traditional and modern providers. The focus of this chapter is primarily upon the modern, for-profit sector, as it is this sector which is most often discussed in relation to a New Public Management strategy to encourage diversity and competition in provision of health care. Where the discussion refers to a different part of the health sector this is explicitly stated. Most of the measures examined focus upon the regulation and enabling of private health services (i.e. provision) not financing. Although in India and Zimbabwe, regulation and liberalisation of private health insurance was an important policy area, this was not the focus of the field research.[1] It is commonly said that regulation may address the prices, quantity or quality of health services (Maynard 1982). Quite which of these variables government is interested in addressing will influence the type of measures adopted. In practice, very few of the regulatory or enabling measures encountered in study countries focused upon price: most were concerned with the quantity and quality of private health services.

Table 7.1 Measures to enable and regulate the private sector

Policy type	Potential measures
Liberalisation policies	• Repeal or relax laws prohibiting private practice for various cadres • Permit public sector doctors to do private practice • Permit private practitioners to admit patients to public hospitals • Break monopoly on purchasing from public sector pharmaceutical companies or distributors • Repeal laws prohibiting private health insurance
Enabling policies	• Increase technical support to private sector (such as training activities, dissemination of guidelines) • Provide incentives for improved performance (such as accreditation) • Provide financial subsidies through low interest loans or tax holidays • Make credit for private health sector more accessible • Reform health care finance so as to facilitate use of private providers
Regulation	• Implement laws requiring registration of private providers (including clinics, hospitals, pharmacies, diagnostic centres) • Set or raise standards required of private providers • Increase strength of regulatory bodies through increased funding, enhanced status, or strengthened information systems • Facilitate processes to prosecute private providers in cases of malpractice or negligence • Increase support and monitoring of professional regulatory bodies, such as medical councils • Implement or strengthen regulation regarding establishment of private medical schools
Information provision	• Monitoring of structural and process aspects of private services, and provision of information to general public on services

The following sections review the specific policy context for reform in the area of enabling and regulating in the case study countries, review current policies in this area and examine the extent to which policies were turned into practice. Government performance of enabling and regulatory measures is assessed, and government capacity to be effective in this area examined.

2. The policy context in study countries

2.1 Development of the private health sector

International literature about appropriate directions for development of government policy on the private health sector tends to start from the potential advantages of expanding private health care delivery; however, actual experience in the study countries indicated a rather different starting point. In all three of the Asian countries (India, Sri Lanka and Thailand), rapid growth in the private health sector had occurred during the 1980s and early 1990s (Bhat 1999, Nittayaramphong and Tangchar-oensathien 1994). This growth was generally not due to the direct effects of liberalisation or enabling policies implemented by the Ministry of Health, and in all three cases, it was at least partially attributable to perceptions of poor quality public sector care. In Thailand, for example, long queues, poor hotel aspects of care and sometimes physical inaccessibility of outpatient departments of public hospitals had encouraged people increasingly to use private providers. In India, very poor standards of hygiene and high informal payments in the public sector had had similar effects.

Although there were clearly other determinants of private sector growth apart from the price, quality and accessibility of public sector services, including the regulatory environment and community perceptions of private sector quality, the dominant explanatory factor in the study countries appeared to be the macro-economic context. Rapid income growth in Thailand had led to a private sector boom (at least prior to the recent economic collapse), and in India and Sri Lanka pockets of economic growth had encouraged private sector expansion.

The macro-economic situation in Sub-Saharan Africa had been much more adverse than that seen in Asia, and correspondingly the market for private health services had remained smaller. In Ghana there was a relatively large private ambulatory care sector (for example over 40 per cent of health centres were reportedly private for-profit), but most providers were concentrated in the traditional and informal sectors. Zimbabwe had one of the larger private health sectors in Sub-Saharan Africa, which had emerged after Independence in 1980. In the four years preceding the research there had been rapid private sector development and a growing number of people taking up private health insurance. This growth was probably due partly to government policies, but also to declining quality in the public health sector resulting from economic recession.

2.2   Key policy actors

Of the four policies studied in this research, the issue of regulation and enabling has perhaps the most complex set of policy actors. The key types of actor, and the specific bodies in one of the study settings, Tamil Nadu, are described in Table 7.2. The primary interests of these actors are also

Table 7.2   Key policy actors on regulatory and enabling issues in Tamil Nadu

Type	Specific actors	Interests
Government	**Policy-makers** Department of Health/State **Implementing agencies** e.g. Drug Control Authority	Implement policies to ensure basic minimum quality of private sector care Protect business interests Implement government policy *Preserve livelihoods of inspectors through abuse of regulatory authority (e.g. charging 'back-handers')*
Statutory Regulatory Bodies	Tamil Nadu Medical Council TN Nursing Council TN Homeopathic Council Indian Medicine Council Pharmacy Council	Ensure that behaviour of members meets standards set out by the Council and/or government *Protect and represent interests of members of profession*
Providers	**Private** • formal/informal • for-profit/non-profit • provider organisations (e.g. Independent Medical Practitioners Association) **Public** e.g. TN Government Doctors' Association	Protect business interests: whether these are of full-time private practitioners or part-time private practitioners (who are also likely to hold a government post)
Legal	Judiciary and Consumer Protection Courts	Protect patients against malpractice and negligence in both public and private sectors
Civil Society	Consumer organisations e.g. Federation of Consumer Organisations of Tamil Nadu	Represent consumer interests in policy and protect consumer rights under the law

shown. In the area of regulation and enabling, it is particularly the case that in addition to formal, explicit interests which actors express, they also commonly have informal interests. These are shown in italics in Table 7.2. As these informal interests tended not to be articulated it is difficult to describe them with certainty, but a considerable amount of anecdotal evidence suggested that such interests were present in Tamil Nadu.

Amongst these actors there were multiple principal–agent relationships: for example, statutory regulatory bodies represented government in

enforcing certain aspects of regulation, consumer organisations represented consumers in policy discussion and might legally represent
consumers in courts. Savedoff (1998) observes that situations where
multiple principals rely on one agent to represent their interests are
particularly problematic as it is then very difficult to structure incentive
mechanisms which encourage the agent to pursue multiple interests.
Several such cases of multiple principals being represented by one agent
exist in health care regulation: for example, government policy-makers
need to represent the interests of both consumers and business; statutory
regulatory bodies might represent the interests of both consumers and
health care professionals. These principal–agent relationships are made
even more complex because some of them are informal and unarticulated.
For example, medical councils are generally not supposed to represent the
interests of the medical profession – although they are commonly accused
of so doing.

Formal and informal interests very commonly conflict. This is clearly
the case for inspection agencies given the responsibility of implementing
regulations. The rights associated with the implementation of regulation
may be misused so that inspectors pursue their own interests (as when
they accept a bribe in return for not reporting a substandard facility)
rather than maintain quality standards.

The relative strengths of the different actors listed in Table 7.2 varied
significantly between countries studied: for example, the situation in
India was perhaps notable for the strength of civil society organisations
and the judiciary. In all cases, however, physicians as a group had played a
particularly influential role in the development of regulatory and
enabling policy. This power seemed to stem not only from their critical
inputs into the process of health care delivery, but also from the generally
high regard in which they were held by society. For example, in
Zimbabwe, where doctors were scarce, it was suggested that authorities
were reluctant to deregister doctors and therefore were particularly
cautious about how they handled this lobby. However, even in India
where the number of physicians per capita was three times higher (see
Table 2.1), physicians had exerted considerable influence by virtue of
their position in society, and had often used this influence to retard the
development of regulation.

In all the study countries except Ghana, public doctors were allowed to
do private practice.[2] In Sri Lanka and Thailand, the majority of doctors in
private practice also held public sector posts. This practice had led to a
number of complexities in the way in which public and private sectors
related and exacerbated problems of conflict between formal, articulated

and informal, unarticulated interests. For example, public sector doctors in Sri Lanka commonly worked in private 'channelling clinics'. They received a decent fee for this work but also referred to themselves in public hospitals (or private hospitals if patients could afford it). Elsewhere (and more commonly), government doctors were reported to refer the wealthier patients whom they saw in the public sector to their private practices.

Such public–private cross-over arrangements appeared more problematic in some countries than others. For example in India, many doctors will work only a couple of hours in the government facility in the morning before proceeding to their private practice whereas in Thailand, government doctors tended to practice privately in evening hours and there was not the same abuse of government position. It was difficult to explain these variations. While there were certainly some differences in the consistency with which staff in Thailand and India were monitored, informal rules or institutions probably played a more critical role. For example, in Sri Lanka, it was thought that private doctors took considerable pride in their profession and maintained reasonably close contact with the MOH, which might have prevented some of the worst examples of malpractice, and induced demand, such as those reported in India.

In addition to the actors centrally involved in regulation, donors appeared to be increasingly inclined to address regulatory topics. The World Bank (an influential donor in India) had clearly recognised the central importance of more effective regulation:

> The main issue with private practising doctors in India is that there is a wide array of qualified and less than qualified practitioners. Most are unregistered, unlicensed and unregulated. (The World Bank, 1994)

2.3   Recent policy trends

In the Asian countries, it appeared that the Ministries of Health had for many years been positively uninterested in regulatory issues and policy on the private sector. Consequently, private sector expansion had occurred in a policy vacuum with no concurrent reforms to ensure adequate quality. For example, in India, until recently, registration of private providers had been required only in four states. The Board of Investment in Thailand had run a tax subsidy scheme throughout the 1980s, offering substantial incentives to private sector investment in health, in which the Ministry of Public Health had played virtually no role.

By the time of the study, in all three Asian countries, there was substantial dependence upon private sector provision of care (see Table 2.3) and the policy environment was not pushing towards liberalisation but rather towards improving quality amongst private providers and obtaining more information about them. During the previous couple of years, policy statements in each of these countries had been made with this aim in mind. The policy stances sounded remarkably similar despite differences in the context:

> facilitate the development and regulation of the private health care sector and promote better co-ordination within the sector. (Ministry of Health, Sri Lanka, National Health Policy, 1996)

> strengthen the co-ordination and mobilisation of health resources for development, from for-profit private sector and non-profit private sector and general population to participate in health development. (Ministry of Public Health, Thailand, Seventh Five year National Health Development Plan, 1992)

Whilst in private, health officials had recognised substantial problems with the way in which the private sector was operating, official policy documents spoke much more of coordination and partnerships rather than regulation. For example, the Sri Lankan government had framed its objective as developing and guiding the private sector and the new regulatory unit established in the Ministry of Health had been called the 'Private Sector Development Unit'.

In Ghana, the government had banned private practice by government medical officers in 1960, so those doctors who had entered private practice were those whose foreign qualifications were less preferred by government. This effectively gave private practice a poor reputation which it had never quite shaken off. Recent policy statements, like those in Asia, had talked about the need for improved coordination:

> in the medium term, partnerships between public and private providers of health care will be actively promoted. (Ministry of Health, Ghana, Medium Term Health Strategy, 1995)

None the less specific proposals under this strategy seemed to have focused much more on regulation and quality control than 'partnerships'.

In Zimbabwe the need for regulation had been more openly admitted. The Health Reform Agenda (MOHCW 1996) had stated that regulatory mechanisms were needed to implement accreditation of private providers, to control technological and capital investment, monitor private sector health care financing, and strengthen the Health Professions Council (Hongoro et al. 1998).

Perhaps more than was the case for any of the other policy areas examined in this research, policy in the area of regulation and enabling had commonly been made either unintentionally or by actors outside of the health sector. For example, policies most successful at promoting private sector growth had sometimes been the inadvertent consequence of policy changes in health financing. In Thailand, the establishment of the Social Security Scheme, and rules under the scheme allowing beneficiaries to seek care from the private sector, had considerably boosted demand at some private hospitals and encouraged further investment. In Sri Lanka, private practice by government doctors had been deregulated in 1976/7 with the aims of discouraging public sector physicians from leaving the country and encouraging doctors to remain in rural areas; this had contributed significantly to private sector growth.

Finally, the links between private sector growth and broader macro-economic and industrial policy were strong. In Sri Lanka, an economic liberalisation framework implemented by the government in 1977 had increased the availability of capital by the mid-1980s, making purchase of medical equipment and pharmaceutical imports much easier, and thus lowering barriers to private practice. The Board of Investment in Sri Lanka had also encouraged foreign investment in the private health sector through a variety of incentive schemes. In Thailand, overall government policy had been very supportive of the private sector, and the Board of Investment had provided subsidies to private hospital companies.

3.   Policy measures implemented

This section documents the recent policy changes which had occurred in the case study countries and, where possible, the forces which had helped to bring about these changes.

3.1   Liberalisation and enabling

Liberalisation had not been a key feature of the reforms in the study countries because the private sector was already substantial, and a fairly liberal set of policies had existed. Recent liberalising measures had addressed relatively small parts of the health system which had previously been overlooked. For example, in Ghana, a proposed new Act would formally allow nurses to own and operate private practices; previously only doctors had been permitted to do so, although many had effectively been run by nurses. In India, liberalisation of private health insurance under the Insurance Regulatory Authority Bill had been planned but was not yet approved by parliament at the time of the research. This bill would effectively liberalise all forms of insurance, but the liberalisation process would start in the health insurance sector. Liberalisation of insurance had been part of one of the policies included in the structural adjustment package agreed with the World Bank, and the central government had proceeded with it against the wishes of the Department of Health.

Although several countries had mentioned certain 'enabling' measures as part of recent policy, few of these appeared to have actually been implemented. Most of the enabling measures in place stemmed from (i) long-standing historical relationships, (ii) piecemeal efforts (often supported by donors) to encourage private sector participation in a certain field, or (iii) policies initiated outside of the health sector. Thus these measures had had little connection with New Public Management as applied to the health sector, or with the envisaged new roles of government. Perhaps a partial exception to this was India where there had been several recent efforts to enable greater or more structured private sector participation in health care delivery. Several of these interventions were fairly innovative in nature and did adhere to NPM precepts; however they were largely donor-supported, and had remained on a very small scale compared both to traditional public and private sectors. Table 7.3 summarises the enabling measures identified in the study countries.

Policy pronouncements, particularly in Ghana and Zimbabwe, had suggested that more innovative NPM-type enabling measures to encourage private sector participation were planned. For example, the Medium Term Health Strategy in Ghana discussed public–private partnerships and in particular proposed:

- to provide incentives and support to private providers to enable them to offer a basic package of health services and to attract them into areas without government health services;
- to establish a common framework for policy development, planning and evaluation for both public and private sectors.

However, at the time of the research no measures had been undertaken to implement either of these policy proposals. In Zimbabwe the fairly radical plans for a purchaser/provider split (see Chapter 6) would also enable the

Table 7.3 Existing enabling measures in study countries

Type of measure	Countries with measure	Measures
Historical support to non-profit providers or charitable cases	Ghana Zimbabwe	Grants in kind and cash to members of Church Medical Association (Ghana and Zimbabwe)
	India	Tax breaks to private hospitals guaranteeing a proportion of beds for indigent patients and free services for these patients (applies to both for-profit and non-profit providers in India)
Programme-specific initiatives	Ghana	Free vaccines to private providers complying with certain standards Subsidised family planning supplies (from USAID) Training for members of Ghana Registered Midwives Association (USAID)
Centrally-initiated tax breaks, preferential loans, etc.	Zimbabwe	Tax-exempt status given to Medical Aid Societies, tax credits for employer and employee contributions to medical insurance schemes
	India	Loans at concessional rates for private hospitals, tax-breaks on imports; arrangements varied by state
	Sri Lanka	Tax-breaks for private hospitals, medical imports tax-free, sales tax exemption for medical services, Board of Investment tax breaks, import duty exemptions and waiver of labour laws for foreign firms investing in health care
	Thailand	Board of Investment support (tax-breaks and waivers on import duties)

Source for Zimbabwe data: Mudyarabikwa (1999).

purchase of care from the private sector. However, like the plans in Ghana, this had been proposed but not yet implemented.

In India the size of the private sector, and its importance in service provision, had meant that many external analysts had sought ways to enable the private sector to offer more and better quality care. For example, the World Health Organisation had supported initiatives to set up franchising arrangements with the private sector for TB control. In Delhi, a joint partnership between Apollo Hospitals Co. and the government of the Union Territory of Delhi had been planned (with support from the International Finance Corporation) to establish a new

Table 7.4 Key regulatory statutes in study countries

Country	Regulations governing hospitals/ nursing homes	Regulations governing individuals	Regulations governing pharmaceuticals
Ghana	Private Hospitals and Maternity Homes Act (1958) provided for registration and inspection of private facilities. Allowed Board to set standards (however standards had not been specified)	Medical and Dental Council and Nurses and Midwives Council had been established with responsibility for registering practitioners and regulating professional education. Several allied health professions (e.g. laboratory medicine and the traditional sector) remained unregulated.	Previous duplication (through Pharmacy and Drugs Act 1961 and Ghana Standards Board) resolved through the recent Pharmacy Council Bill separating regulation of pharmacy practice and drug control and also establishment of new Food and Drugs Board.
Zimbabwe	Medical Dental and Allied Professions Act (1971 plus several further amendments) – registration of all health institutions in accordance with defined structural minimum standards	Medical Dental and Allied Professions Act (1971 plus further amendments) provided for establishment of Health Professions Council (HPC) and registration of all health professionals with this Council (except natural therapists and traditional practitioners who had their own). Allowed monitoring and control of practice standards and inspection of training institutions	Drugs and Allied Substances Act (1969) established Drug Control Council responsible for drug registration, licensing, control and inspection of pharmacies and regulation of clinical trials
India (Tamil Nadu)	TN Private Clinical Establishments Act (1997) (passed but not implemented) provided for establishment of regulatory authority, compulsory registration (every five years) of all facilities with beds, and set structural standards	Madras Medical Registration Act (1914), Madras Nurses and Midwives Act (1925) and similar for other professions: established professional council, controlled medical education, individual registration. Plus similar All India Acts. Tort law for medical negligence claims	All India 1940 Drug Act (amended as The Drug and Cosmetic Act) covered import, manufacture and sale of pharmaceuticals

Table 7.4 *(continued)*

Country	Regulations governing hospitals/ nursing homes	Regulations governing individuals	Regulations governing pharmaceuticals
Sri Lanka	Nursing Homes Regulation Act 1949, Ayurveda Act 1961, Homeopathy Act 1970 each allowed for registration and quality monitoring of facilities offering these different types of care	Medical Ordinances Act, Ayurveda Act and Homeopathy Act allowed for establishment of professional Council, control of professional education, and individual registration for each of these professions	The Cosmetic Devices and Drugs Act 1980/84 established technical advisory committee and licensing for manufacturers, importers and retailers, plus quality controls. Opiums and Dangerous Drugs Act prohibited dangerous drugs, set standards of strength, etc. Consumer Protection Act safeguarded public from unscrupulous sales including drugs
Thailand	Medical Institutions Act (1961) provided for annual registration, definition of standards, inspection, provision of information to MOPH and prohibited false advertising	Medical Professionals Act 1982, Nursing and Midwife Professionals Act and similar for other professions, established professional councils, controlled professional education and registered individuals	Pharmacist professionals act provided for pharmacy council and registration of individuals. Food and Drug Administration Act provided powers to register, monitor and inspect drug manufacturers, wholesalers and retailers

tertiary hospital. A recently completed loan by the World Bank to the health sector had provided financial incentives for state governments to involve the private sector in delivery of certain priority services such as HIV control and prevention. This had resulted in the establishment of private non-profit societies such as the Tamil Nadu State Aids Control Society.

3.2   Regulatory measures

As Table 7.4 indicates, all the study countries (with the partial exception of India) had in place a fairly substantial regulatory framework governing whom might practice different aspects of medicine, where they might practice it (in terms of the standards of medical facilities), and the importation, manufacture, wholesale and retail of drugs. India was notable in that at the beginning of 1997, only three states (Maharastra, Karnataka and the Union Territory of Delhi) had legislation requiring the registration of private hospitals and allowing for inspection of such facilities.

In addition to the key regulatory laws noted in the table, most countries had a variety of other forms of regulation which had affected the health sector to some extent, such as the regulation of insurance markets. None of the countries appeared to have had restrictions on the importation or use of high-technology medical equipment. Despite the substantive nature of existing health sector regulations, all of the core study countries were engaged in fairly far-reaching regulatory reforms, in general because existing regulations had evolved over a long period of time, and were thought to be duplicative, labyrinthine and subject to a number of loopholes.

In Ghana a new bill had been drafted to replace the outdated Private Hospitals and Maternity Homes Act (1958). This new bill:

- required the annual renewal of licenses for all private hospitals and maternity homes;
- allowed the Private Hospitals and Maternity Homes Board to specify standards for premises;
- extended regulatory oversight to laboratory and nursing practices;
- established regional inspectorates.

The Ghanaian government had also recently passed a new bill covering the pharmaceutical sector (the Pharmacy Council Bill) which replaced the 1961 Pharmacy and Drugs Act. The new bill had separated the functions of regulating pharmaceutical production and drugs control and established new regulatory bodies to cover these two distinct areas, though had only been partially implemented. The Ghanaian government at the time of the research had proposed a number of further regulatory reforms, particularly to cover a variety of hitherto unregulated health professionals (dietetics, laboratory medicine, physiotherapy).

In Zimbabwe, several recent reforms had been undertaken to strengthen the regulatory framework. Recent amendments to the Medical, Dental and Allied Professions Act had required (i) that every health practitioner and health institution provide relevant information pertaining to any allegation of improper conduct or incompetence (1993 amendment), and (ii) that the Health Professions Council take over the registration and inspection of private health facilities from local government bodies. Furthermore, the 1997 Medical Services Bill (which at the time of the research had been gazetted but not passed by parliament) had expanded the Minister of Health's regulatory powers to encompass the price of care in all state-aided hospitals, referrals between private and public sectors, and private non-profit insurance organisations called Medical Aid Societies (which had hitherto been unregulated).

Statutes providing for regulation of the private health sector in India were probably weaker than in the other countries studied. The situation was made more complex by the fact that most regulatory statutes were issued at the state level and hence there was substantial variation from state to state. A meeting in January 1997 of the Central Council of Health and Welfare had concluded that a large number of private and voluntary hospitals were being operated without adequate staff, equipment or infrastructure. The conference had urged state governments to enact laws to provide for registration of only those private hospitals with adequate facilities (Government of India 1997). The state assembly of Tamil Nadu had approved such a bill just a couple of weeks later and some other states had passed similar legislation during 1997. However, at the time of the research none had succeeded in properly implementing the new laws. Several factors helped explain this including the very strong interest groups in India, many of which had opposed stricter regulation; difficulties encountered in setting standards which could be applied to facilities serving communities with widely disparate income levels; and the organisational structure of Departments of Health which generally had no distinct body responsible for regulation.

The second measure relevant to regulatory reform in the Indian context was the extension of the Consumer Protection Act to cover medical care provided for a fee (1992) and later its further extension to cover any services provided in a facility which had charged any patient a fee (1995). The latter ruling was significant as it had essentially brought free care at government hospitals under the Act. Consumer courts had made action under tort law much more accessible since cases going to the civil courts were expensive and generally extremely time-consuming, often taking twenty years to reach a conclusion (Advani 1991). In contrast consumer courts were free and cases should be heard and dealt with within a 90 day period. Reform in this area had been effected by the judiciary alone as justices in the courts essentially decided which cases were and were not covered by the Act, and set precedents. While Sri Lanka and Thailand had similar Consumer Protection Acts at the time of the research, neither of these covered medical services, though they did encompass pharmaceuticals.

In Sri Lanka, a new Private Medical Institutions Act had been drafted to replace the outdated Nursing Homes Act. This new Act should improve upon the old in a number of respects. First, it would widen the coverage of the legislation to apply to all private medical institutions including small private clinics. Second, it aimed to formulate a system of quality assurance, and an accreditation scheme might at a later stage be formulated and enforced. Third, private facilities would be graded to provide users with information about the services they offered and quality of these services and fourthly, the Advisory Council to be established under the Act should provide a forum for better coordination of public and private sectors. While the Act had been drafted a few years previously, it had not, at the time of the research, been submitted to Parliament. The National Health Advisory Committee which had formulated the Act was particularly aware of the importance of strong implementation, through regular and systematic surveillance procedures. Consequently a new Division within the MOH, headed by a new Director of Private Medical Sector Development, had already been established.

4.   Performance of liberalisation, enabling and regulatory measures

4.1   Liberalisation and enabling

Liberalisation, or one time change in rules, appeared to have been performed effectively where there had been changes, though there had been very little monitoring or evaluation of the effects of liberalisation. One survey of private practices in Ghana had noted that only 7 per cent of respondents had said that regulations had been a problem in starting their clinic (Private Initiatives for Primary Health Care 1995).

Despite policy pronouncements about desirable enabling measures in several countries (such as Ghana and Zimbabwe), these had not at the time of the research been implemented. Instead, as suggested in the previous sections, existing measures appeared largely piecemeal and donor-driven (as in Ghana), or initiated and implemented by bodies outside of the health sector.

The most substantive evidence about government performance with respect to enabling measures concerned the implementation of subsidies and tax-breaks aimed at promoting private sector growth in India and Thailand. This evidence highlighted a number of problems in performance. Criteria as to who were eligible to receive subsidies or tax-breaks were commonly vague, inappropriate or difficult to verify. In India, hospitals reserving 10 per cent of beds for indigent patients and providing free care to these patients were entitled to tax-breaks. However, it had proved very difficult to verify that hospitals were actually meeting these criteria and private hospitals had been accused of abusing the law by providing free care to politicians, staff and relatives of staff who were not actually indigent. Evidence from elsewhere also suggests that lack of clarity in criteria for awarding subsidies results in clientelism: in Venezuela, for example, subsidies for private non-profit health care providers were distributed by politicians who had limited knowledge of the health sector and received no technical advice; their decisions were observed to be both erratic and frequently in favour of their own interests (Werna 1995).

Incentives were often poorly coordinated with the rest of the health system. For example, for many years the Board of Investment (BOI) in Thailand had awarded tax-breaks to any new hospital with 100 beds or more, despite the MOPH's concern about the excess supply of hospital beds in Bangkok. Monitoring of subsidy measures was also generally very weak. In Thailand, although the BOI had started providing tax-breaks to public hospitals in Bangkok in 1974, there was no further monitoring by the MOPH until the early 1990s. The subsidy programme in Venezuela mentioned above was established in the mid-1980s, but it was not until 1994 that measures had been taken to improve grant allocation and ensure that funds were used to meet specified objectives (Werna 1995).

4.2 Regulation

Several country case studies argued that the recent spate of regulatory reform was too little, too late. A patchwork of outdated laws had commonly been in place since the 1940s with (until recently) only minor attempts to update the regulatory framework. Thus laws were often inappropriate. For example:

- in Sri Lanka the 1949 Nursing Homes Regulation Act applied only to nursing homes and hospitals and not to individual private practices or clinics;
- in Ghana medical professions acts did not cover various allied health professionals;
- in Thailand the Medical Institutions Act covered behaviour of medical staff employed by the hospital but not non-medical staff, and hence could not be used to prevent hospital administrators from turning away (even emergency) patients whom they believed were unable to pay hospital fees (locally known as conducting 'wallet biopsies').

Although there were clearly problems with the regulatory frameworks, more serious weaknesses in performance were evident with respect to the implementation of regulations. Country case studies were virtually unanimous on the weak implementation of regulation: both regulatory councils and Ministries of Health had performed poorly. As Table 7.4 indicated, most of the regulation related to the process aspects of care had been delegated to professional councils. Such self-regulation appeared to have been very ineffective. Medical and professional councils had tended to adopt very passive approaches to regulation, failing to inform the general public of their role and waiting for consumers to bring complaints to them. Consequently such councils had played a minimal role in controlling poor conduct by professionals. For example, in Ghana, the last case of medical malpractice heard by the medical council had been ten years previously. In Tamil Nadu, only four or five cases of malpractice came before the council each year and within the previous ten years only one doctor had been struck off the list. In Maharastra state in India, during the past 30 years only three doctors had been deregistered (one for murdering his wife and two for inappropriate advertising).

While in most instances the performance of professional councils was characterised principally by inactivity, or at worst a certain protectionism, in India Medical Councils had been accused of corruption. For example, in Maharastra state in 1992, a number of members had stood for election stating that they would 'clean up' the Medical Council. Subsequent reports had suggested that there was substantial vote-rigging during the elections in order to prevent any of the reforming doctors being elected (Jesani 1996). Many critics had claimed publicly that the Medical Council of India had approved licences for medical colleges on the basis of 'personal favours' or hospitality offered by the owners despite the facilities clearly not meeting set standards.

The very poor performance by professional councils in all the study countries could be partially attributed to weak supervision by Ministries of Health. For example in Tamil Nadu, senior Department of Health officials had no knowledge of the composition of the Medical Council. However, despite the generally bleak picture with respect to the performance of professional councils, there were a handful of counter-examples such as that in Box 7.1.

Government performance with respect to the implementation of regulation had also showed many weaknesses. For example, one of the most basic aspects of regulation is the maintenance of a database of private providers, which then acts as reference for all further regulatory efforts. In all four core countries, data on the number and location of private health care providers were highly incomplete. In Thailand this most basic of measures was implemented effectively.

Box 7.1   The Nurses and Midwives Council of Ghana

One exception to the rule of poor performance by professional councils was the Nurses and Midwives Council in Ghana which both set registration standards and was involved in curriculum development and examinations. The Council had the reputation for being both highly motivated and very proactive. It employed 37 staff in all including 10 professionals. It was funded by a subvention from the MOH and since 1995 had been able to retain revenue from registration.

Lack of funds had affected the ability of the Council to inspect training institutions spread throughout the country, but it had tried to counter this by developing guidelines which could then be used by local health officials to whom were delegated the responsibility of inspecting. Since funding constraints meant they had no transport of their own, Council staff used public transport.

Whilst the Council had a high reputation, it seemed that they were not fully enforcing current regulations. Nurses were not allowed to own and run their own private practice in Ghana but it would seem that this regulation was widely flouted.

It was difficult to explain the superior performance of this particular Council over other professional councils in Ghana. The nursing profession was generally perceived to have a stronger collective orientation and greater concern with maintaining standards than other professions. In addition the Council had drawn strength from a programme of information exchange with UK counterparts.

Often legislation specified merely that the Ministry of Health had the right to set standards and actual standards had then to be formulated. Several governments had encountered difficulty in doing this. In Mumbai, standards required under the 1949 Nursing Home Act had, at the time of the research, not been agreed. In 1991 a commission was established to agree standards for the Mumbai municipal area, but this commission had failed to make progress. Disagreement often arose over the relevance of structural standards: while these are the easiest to measure, they may have very little impact upon quality of care. In Thailand the standards had emphasised structural quality – particularly infrastructure (e.g. number of square metres per bed, number of toilets available) but had not addressed other aspects of quality, such as staffing, which may have been much more critical to quality of care.

Regulatory units within Ministries of Health had failed to inspect routinely the private facilities which were registered. For example, in Mumbai, the inspection authorities had admitted that they had not visited facilities in several wards for two to three years (India Today 1995). A contrasting example came from Sri Lanka, where a central MOH official had been given responsibility for identifying staff who were carrying out private practice during public working hours. Although only one or two people had been punished for this each year, it at least provided some disincentive to abuse public posts.

The various examples cited above demonstrated weaknesses in the way in which regulations had been formulated and implemented. Had these weaknesses adversely affected the quality of care of private sector health services? While there was a lack of well-designed studies on this topic, there was considerable anecdotal evidence to suggest that weak regulation had adversely affected private sector care. There was substantial evidence of the private sector providing care of an unacceptable standard in India (Uplekar 1989a and 1989b): this was partly due to providers lacking up-to-date information about appropriate diagnosis and treatment but also providers had consciously skimped on care (or overprovided certain profitable services) in order to make more money. In Thailand several high-profile cases had occurred where patients in a critical condition had been turned away from hospital due to their perceived inability to pay for care. These incidents would most likely have been averted if regulations had been more effective. In Ghana there had been general concern at the uncontrolled importation and sale of drugs with reports of substandard ampicillin injections from India reaching the market. While these problems were indicative of weak government performance, they must be interpreted in the light of common perceptions of poor quality public sector care described in Chapter 2.

5.   Government capacity to regulate and enable

5.1   Internal aspects of capacity

Lack of funds and lack of staff were commonly cited as problems impeding effective regulation; this was the case in all four core countries studied. For example, in Tamil Nadu in 1996, there were a total of 87 drug inspectors in the state who were supposed to cover 2,800 manufacturers of drugs and cosmetics, 11,500 licensed sales outlets and an unknown (but probably larger still) number of unlicensed sales outlets. Similarly in Sri Lanka the Drug Regulatory Authority (DRA) had only 25 inspectors – one for each district. The head of the DRA had noted that access to vehicles and per diems to improve inspection coverage was limited by resource constraints. In Ghana, just four drug inspectors were supposed to cover the entire Greater Accra area. In Sri Lanka there used to be 'no unit or staff within the MOH responsible for registration, monitoring or co-ordination of private providers, at any level of the organisation' (Russell and Attanayake 1997). Low salaries had compounded the problem of limited staff. Low salaries not only adversely affected staff motivation but, as was noted in Sri Lanka, may encourage the acceptance of bribes in order to allow registration of a particular facility or prevent it being closed.

The limited amount of resources available for regulation may have been partially due to the fact that regulation was (at least until recently) rarely seen as a priority function for government in the health sector. In Thailand, for example, the licensing division of the MOPH had only very recently been computerised, but other departments within the Ministry had made extensive use of computers for many years. This situation may be changing as regulatory issues attract greater attention. The establishment of a new regulatory unit in Sri Lanka headed by dynamic, young officials may signal a sea change.

More specific skills or systems within government which case studies had identified as necessary for effective regulatory performance but which were currently lacking included lack of legal expertise to help draft regulatory reform bills (Ghana) and inadequate information systems (which was a widespread problem). Government collection of data from the private health sector was made more difficult by the inadequacy of records kept by private providers. Government needed to address this problem of private sector record-keeping before it could substantially improve its own information systems on the private sector.

As the discussion has highlighted, professional councils were generally the key actors involved in regulating process aspects of care, but had often performed this task very poorly. Lack of resources within professional councils was problematic in some contexts: for example in Maharastra state, it was said that the Medical Council relied on 'minimal' grants from government (Jesani 1996). In Zimbabwe lack of staffing at the Health Professions Council was widely perceived to be a key explanatory factor for its poor performance. But lack of resources was by no means the rule. In Tamil Nadu fees paid by physicians registering with the Council were fairly substantial and should have provided sufficient resources for a stronger regulatory function than that played by the Council.

It was sometimes said that medical councils lacked autonomy from government and that this contributed to their ineffectiveness. In Zimbabwe, the Minister of Health and Child Welfare appointed up to one third of council members and this was viewed by some to prevent unbiased and independent decisions. In certain Indian states, government officials occupied many of the seats on Medical Councils. However, this was not the case in all states, and problems still existed in those such as Tamil Nadu where the Medical Council was highly independent of government.

From the case study countries, as well as the broader literature (Allsop and Mulcahy 1996, Moran and Wood 1993), it seemed that the root cause of poor regulatory performance by Medical Councils was inertia, lack of motivation and self-interest. The research unearthed some fairly dramatic examples of how official positions on Medical Councils had been used for private benefit (such as that of inspection of training institutions by the Medical Council of India). More pervasive, however, were instances where Medical Councils had simply protected their own. For example, in Zimbabwe, several respondents had expressed concern that the physician-dominated Health Professions Council heard all malpractice and negligence cases *in camera* and never publicised the results of such cases.

Some analysts have suggested that just as important as the formal channels for regulation are the informal rules and institutions which govern the behaviour of a particular profession (Mackintosh 1997). For example, while formal rules commonly prohibit doctors to whom referrals are made paying a cut of the fee back to the referring doctor, in certain contexts informal norms widely support this practice (Yesudian 1994). In most of the study countries the medical profession had clearly formed a fairly tight-knit group with its own professional culture; only in a few places, such as Sri Lanka, did this culture seem to have reinforced behaviour conducive to high standards of medical practice. Often, instead, informal rules had protected the profession at the expense of the patient. For example, under the Consumer Protection Act in India, it had proved very difficult to get doctors to testify against others as this was viewed as breaking the professional bond between them.

5.2 Coordination between actors

Of all the policy areas considered in this research, regulation involves the most complex issues of coordination between different actors. This complexity stems from the variety of complementary approaches to regulation which need to fit together. Several country case studies emphasised the capacity weaknesses due to poor coordination. In Tamil Nadu, communication between the Department of Health and the various statutory self-regulatory bodies had appeared almost non-existent. Under the Tamil Nadu Medical Council Act, the Council had no responsibility to report any of its operations to the Department of Health. In Ghana, considerable confusion had sprung from the former division of responsibilities between the Pharmacy Board and the Ghana Standards Board, both of whom had borne some responsibility for pharmaceutical regulation.

Decentralisation can have implications for the effective coordination of regulatory functions. In Sri Lanka, responsibilities for regulatory functions were unclear after decentralisation to the provinces in 1988. The central Drug Regulatory Authority could no longer directly intervene in pharmaceutical regulation at the provincial level but was given an advisory role. Responsibility for implementing the Nursing Homes Act was transferred to the provinces without any new guidance. In Zimbabwe, recent regulatory amendments had surprisingly transferred the responsibility for inspecting and registering private health care establishments from local government to the (centrally organised) Health Professions Council (HPC), although the thrust of most other reforms taking place was to promote greater decentralisation. The new arrangement had proved problematic as the HPC did not have the capacity to conduct inspections. Subsequently, an informal agreement between local authorities and the HPC had been reached whereby local authorities would continue to carry out inspections and forward their recommendations to the HPC for final approval.

The federal nature of Indian government had also posed challenges to effective regulation. Regulatory statutes differed from state to state and doctors struck off the list in one state might freely practise in another. Each state had a medical council in addition to the overall Medical Council of India (MCI): communication between the MCI and state medical councils appeared weak.

5.3 External factors affecting capacity

In several countries, but particularly the Asian ones, delayed response by government to issues emerging from growth of the private sector had allowed significant private sector interest groups to develop which tended to oppose tighter regulation. Private sector providers were frequently very influential actors. This stemmed partly from their wealth (investors in hospitals tended to be very affluent) and status (many private sector investors were doctors and gained status by virtue of their profession). But the case studies also highlighted the problems of the permeable boundaries between public and private sectors since in India, Sri Lanka, Thailand and Zimbabwe government doctors all engaged extensively in private practice. Reluctance to enforce private sector regulation was often identified with fear of confrontation with public sector employees. For example in Sri Lanka, the Government Medical Officers Association had called all government consultants out on strike in protest against a proposal to make doctors choose between working in public and private sectors (ie. to prohibit dual practice). Only in Ghana did the private sector not seem to constitute a powerful lobby, possibly because few government doctors carried out private practice and private doctors were in the minority in the Medical Association.

Private sector actors may be backed by the power of big business and multinationals. This is particularly true of the pharmaceutical sector, where there is much evidence of the ineffectiveness of regulatory authorities against such actors. In Maharastra, a new Commissioner of the state drug control authority had started proceedings against several pharmaceutical companies (including a number of well-known multinationals) for selling sub-standard products to a wholesaler in the knowledge that they would then be resold on the black market. The commissioner was suddenly and inexplicably transferred to the state co-operative marketing federation (Pandya 1994).

The broader legal, social and cultural context can also be important in determining the effectiveness of government legislation. In Sri Lanka, the imbalance was marked between weak consumer protection under the law, a poorly organised consumer sector and very weak consumer voice compared to the organised medical profession. In contrast, in India the consumer movement had become increasingly active and had helped to bring health care under the remit of the Consumer Protection Act. Similarly in Zimbabwe, users had formed a powerful lobby for stronger regulation. NGOs can be powerful allies to government in ensuring effective regulation: they can publicise cases where regulatory agencies have been captured, bring transgression of regulatory statutes to government regulatory bodies, support consumer claims, and educate consumers about consumer rights. In India they were playing all of these roles but in the other countries their scope was more limited.

Finally, government capacity to regulate the health sector depends, to no small degree, on how government more broadly is perceived by society: to what extent there is trust and faith in government. The Indian government's own inability to provide health services of an adequate standard had adversely affected its credibility with respect to regulation: private providers thought it laughable that they should be subjected to quality standards which the public sector itself would not meet. This was also true in Zimbabwe where the private sector had questioned how government could regulate quality when quality in the public sector was so low. Where corruption in government is widely prevalent, the costs of implementing regulation may rise significantly. For example, in Tamil Nadu, most private sector providers had thought the 1997 Private Clinical Establishments Act, requiring registration of private hospitals and nursing homes, to be primarily a ruse to generate greater rent-seeking opportunities for government officials. Given such an understanding, it is understandable that private providers had intended to evade the Act, making it considerably more complex and costly for government to implement the regulation.

6.   Conclusions

In the case study countries, regulation and enabling were, at least until recently, very neglected by government. Enabling measures in place had largely originated outside of the sector, or taken the form of very small *ad hoc* measures. Despite the lack of a coherent enabling framework, private sector growth, particularly in the Asian countries, had been rapid. This private sector growth, combined with health sector reforms such as contracting out and decentralisation, had helped to bring regulatory concerns to the forefront of governments' policy agendas. In all four of the core countries there had been a recent flurry of regulatory activity.

While there clearly were loopholes in the legal framework for regulation, weak implementation of existing regulation was a much greater concern – both for the low-income core countries, and in the higher-income reference country. Analysis of the reasons for poor regulatory performance highlighted the inherent difficulty of the regulatory task: in particular the multiplicity of actors involved in regulation, the competing interests of these actors (particularly problematic because of widespread informal, unarticulated interests) and the opacity of information regarding appropriate health care delivery.

With the probable exception of India, the situations described in the core countries studied seemed likely to reflect the prevailing situation in many low income countries. Even in Thailand, a country with a very different cultural context and in some respects considerably greater government capacity than the core countries, problems in enabling and regulation seemed remarkably similar to those encountered in the South Asian core countries with the key exception that stronger government administrative systems meant that the basic data necessary for regulation were available; the problems were thus primarily those of interest group politics.

Some lessons for governments emerge from this analysis. Private sector growth appeared to be influenced more by broader macro-economic conditions than by specific government measures. Hence enabling measures are most useful when the government is attempting to pursue specific goals, such as improving quality of care or enabling private sector services for the poor, rather than the broader objective of achieving private sector growth. Governments need to be very clear and explicit on their enabling goals and this clarity should be reflected in the way enabling measures are formulated. Many of the enabling measures reviewed suffered from very vague criteria which meant that they were open to abuse and clientelism in implementation. There is a dire lack of hard evidence, particularly from low income countries, about the effectiveness of alternative enabling measures under different circumstances. More evaluative work in this area is required to help guide policy.

Formal regulatory measures (such as requiring registration and inspection of private health care establishments) are clearly essential and there are several respects in which governments could strengthen their performance of such measures. For example, databases of private sector providers need to be kept complete and up-to-date. Standards, at the least physical standards, required of private providers need to be clearly specified and enforced. The greater priority which the case study country governments had been recently giving to this area appeared promising. However, such formal regulation appears to work best where regulatory authorities do not have competing and sometimes unarticulated interests, and where there is a strong professional ethos amongst providers. Given the problems described in this chapter, and the evidence from elsewhere of regulatory failure in countries with far greater regulatory capacity, it seems that developing country governments need to pay more attention to the informal rules and norms which govern the behaviour of providers and regulators alike. Measures to help engender a professional ethos which encourages high standards of care and assiduous regulation are probably just as important as the legislative framework. Unfortunately, to date, understanding of how such a professional ethos can be created is very weak.

The substantial private sector role in both the financing and provision of health services in all the study countries, and the evidence (though relatively limited) of poor practice within the private sector, suggests that regulation is a universally important role for governments. However, the substantial weaknesses in government regulation identified here challenge some of the arguments for promoting the private sector which were reviewed at the beginning of this chapter. Many of the theoretical arguments made for promoting the private sector are questionable (Bennett 1997b), and in addition most of them rest upon the existence of an effective regulatory environment. Without such an environment, promoting greater pure private sector involvement in health care may be misguided.

8
Taking Account of Capacity

1. Introduction

The introductory chapter to this book set out a framework for analysing capacity which was used for data collection and analysis in countries. This conceptual framework emphasised:

- *Internal and external aspects of capacity* – the distinction between aspects of capacity internal to the implementing organisation such as the skills and systems present in the Ministry of Health, and external aspects of capacity including the broader political, social and economic environment. It was suggested that development of internal capacity needed to be congruent with the external environment; for example, problems would occur if new financial systems developed by the Ministry of Health did not satisfy government-wide financial regulations.
- *The task-specific nature of capacity* – for example, the capacities required for government to directly finance and deliver health care may be very different from those required for government to contract out services. An assessment of capacity therefore needs to be linked to the tasks to be performed.
- *The dynamic nature of capacity* – capacity is unlikely to remain at a fixed level: it will deteriorate if not invested in and capacities need to be adapted as new systems and tasks emerge. Capacity needs to be adaptive: individuals and organisations must be able to learn from mistakes so as to improve future performance.

The case studies presented in the previous chapters highlight additional dimensions of capacity. Particularly in the Sub-Saharan African countries, reform policies had frequently reached the policy agenda, or even been approved as official government policies, but no further progress had been made in implementation. This was commonly attributable to weaknesses in the process of policy development. It is useful, therefore, to distinguish between the capacity to develop policy and manage the transition, versus the capacity necessary for the day-to-day implementation of the new form of delivery.

Issues concerning the type of capacity constraints prevailing at different levels of the health system were also evident and related to the different tasks which needed to be performed. For example, the nature of capacity problems identified in central Ministries of Health were generally quite different from capacity constraints amongst provider units. None the less these two types of capacity problem were commonly interrelated: inability at the central level to support training or systems development led to continued weak capacity at the provider level.

Overall, the case studies highlighted the complexity of the capacity question. While there were some common conclusions about key capacity constraints which emerged from the case studies, there was also substantial variation by country and by intervention examined. In this context, this chapter aims to:

- summarise key capacity constraints identified in different contexts;
- examine and assess the principal approaches used to overcome such capacity constraints;
- suggest an overall strategy for analysing and addressing capacity in the context of health sector reform programmes.

2. Key capacity constraints

Table 8.1 draws upon the material presented in the previous four chapters to summarise the key capacity constraints faced by governments in designing, preparing and implementing health sector reform programmes containing the four specific policies examined.

2.1 Capacity to design and prepare for reforms

Internal aspects of capacity

For reforms to stand any chance of being successfully implemented, a number of preliminary steps are required: a clear policy framework needs to be developed, commitment to the policy both from internal actors such as health staff and external actors such as politicians needs to be generated, and an implementation strategy needs to be thought through.

Table 8.1 Summary of key capacity constraints

	Designing and preparing for reforms	Implementing new delivery structures
Autonomous hospitals		
Internal	Capacity to develop policy frameworks: lack of attention to detail, especially implementation details. Lack of capacity to improve systems and manage transition. Poor staff motivation to invest in reforms due to low/declining salaries and lack of information about objectives of reform.	Weak basic accounting systems. Weak human resource management systems.
External	Lack of real political commitment to reform stemming partly from lack of ownership of reforms.	Resistance to decentralisation from central-level stakeholders. Corruption due to weak financial controls at lower levels cited as a reason not to decentralise by central level stakeholders. Limited private sector from which to learn new management techniques.
User fees		
Internal	Lack of coherent implementation strategy, due to hurried implementation. Resource constraints in preparing for reform, as implemented at time of economic crisis.	Inappropriate financial incentives for health staff (leading to overcharging or failure to exempt). Weak financial systems for billing and accounting. Weak basic administrative systems. Weak monitoring and supervision by centre. Bureaucracy-wide regulations, e.g. on revenue retention Weak public voice to control provider charging behaviour
External	Economic crisis, and consequently a political environment demanding fast action, prevents adequate planning.	
Contracting		
Internal	Limited capacity to develop policy on contracting due to limited experience with contracting. Health worker resistance to reforms (due to fear of dismissal and sometimes misunderstanding about nature of reform).	Weak information systems (quality and costs) Weak financial systems leading to late payment of contractors

Table 8.1 (*continued*)

	Designing and preparing for reforms	Implementing new delivery structures
External	Lack of political support for reform as benefits not necessarily clear and substantial opposition (especially from workers) implies high political costs.	Civil servant regulations preventing dismissal/ redeployment of staff. Sometimes very limited private sector development (e.g. Sub-Saharan Africa) Overly centralised government-wide management systems Corruption leading to contracts awarded to inefficient contractors
Regulation and enabling		
Internal	Weak incentives to develop effective regulatory framework (public sector actors often have private interests) Lack of legal skills to formulate regulations	Lack of resources: limited funding and staff due partly to low priority given to regulation Lack of adequate information systems on private sector Poor motivation of public sector staff and inappropriate incentives (e.g. inspectors can increase income through accepting bribes and stand little chance of being caught and/or punished) Inadequate communication between large number of actors involved in regulation
External	Vested private sector interests oppose tighter regulation	Private sector organisations resist implementation eg. through failing to register with government Limited government credibility decreases inclination of private sector to comply Corruption accepted as part of political system Public have little voice in system to call for stronger regulation

The central Ministry of Health is often the primary agent responsible for these functions. In several instances, failure to perform effectively one or more of these tasks had suspended the implementation of the reform.

Lack of ability within the MOH to elaborate a policy framework was a commonly perceived problem. The Ghanaian experience with autonomous hospitals was a typical example. After an initial policy statement supporting autonomous hospitals, the MOH had had great difficulty in conceptualising the details of how such a policy would work in practice. Similarly, the lack of experience amongst health staff in Ghana with contracting out services had made it difficult to turn a policy intention into a more detailed policy document. For regulatory policies, a lack of legal skills had commonly impeded the progression from policy intention to detailed policy framework.

Once a clear policy framework is in place, the next necessary step is the development and elaboration of an implementation strategy. All too often this step seemed to have been omitted altogether or given only superficial attention. The lack of an implementation strategy was particularly evident from how user fee policies were handled in Ghana and Zimbabwe.

Finally, garnering support for a policy may be a critical factor in implementation. For several of the policies considered, it was clear that political support was limited and there had been no attempt to communicate the policy to other interest groups (such as health service users) to gain their support. The general public tended to be poorly informed about the nature or purpose of proposed reforms and frequently misunderstood them. For example, in Ghana, community members in focus group discussions had appeared to equate hospital autonomy with some form of privatisation and hence were opposed to it (Rakodi 1996). In none of the case study countries had a proper communication campaign been run to inform the general public of the nature of reforms.

While in most of the countries examined, there were health policy or planning units tasked with the responsibility of developing and elaborating policy, they commonly did not seem to perceive their role in a strategic manner and were preoccupied with the routine business of preparing plans or coordinating with donors. There was a clear lack of capacity in central Ministries of Health to think strategically about policy development and consensus building.

External aspects of capacity

Several of the problems in policy formulation and development stemmed from constraints in the broader environment. As observed earlier, policy change in the two African countries was often agreed upon by a small group of local technicians and external advisors during periods when economic (and to a lesser extent political) crisis was rocking the foundations of government. Under such circumstances, it is hardly surprising that there was frequently no true political commitment to or ownership of reform programmes. If politicians perceived that reforms had been externally imposed, then there was little incentive to give them the public support necessary for success. Similarly, health workers themselves, with a few exceptions such as the user-fee programme in Ghana, did not buy into reform programmes and saw them as externally imposed. This may have substantially reduced their willingness to invest their own personal energies in learning new systems or modes of operation.

This phenomenon of 'policy-making at a time of crisis' often meant that there were unrealistic time-frames for implementation of policies, inhibiting the development of realistic implementation strategies. This was clearly the case for the implementation of user fee policy in Zimbabwe. In addition, economic crises tended to prevent adequate investment in necessary system change and development. Resources available to prepare and disseminate guidelines on the reform, train health staff and make necessary adjustments to existing systems were commonly inadequate.

It is clear from the case studies that economic crisis may create windows of opportunity for reform. Ironically, however, in many instances the crisis also weakens government capacity to plan for and implement change. South African researchers reached a similar conclusion about the mixed blessings created by political windows of opportunity in South Africa:

> A time of radical change in national policy goals has enabled health policy change, but the accompanying change in personnel, govern- ance and administrative structures and macro-economic strategies has also made it exceptionally difficult to develop well-designed policy and to implement policy effectively. (CHP and HEU 1999)

It is primarily those countries where capacity is much stronger to start with which can benefit from these windows of opportunity. For example, the 1997 economic crisis in Thailand had seemed to catalyse action around certain policies which had already been extensively analysed and discussed but had failed to receive the necessary political support for adoption and implementation.

The broader political environment also affected progress in developing and reaching consensus on policy reform. Politicians were often viewed by bureaucrats as unpredictable, making impetuous pronouncements which made rational planning impossible. In Sri Lanka, for example, it was felt that political interference meant that it was difficult to develop a rational reform programme and to commit to implementing policies laid out in the programme:

> politicians make ad hoc decisions, not rational for the health sector, and often change their minds; we have to cope with these decisions. (MOH official quoted in Russell and Attanayake 1997)

The political cycle of elections sometimes affected reform paths. An extreme example of this was found in Zimbabwe where policy on contracting out had been temporarily abandoned by the government during the election period. In contrast in Thailand, there had been multiple changes of government (both democratic and undemocratic) in recent years but the bureaucracy had remained relatively insulated from political changes: broad Enabling Acts were passed by the government and authority for defining the precise content of these acts given to the bureaucracy.

In general, bureaucratic structures did not encourage popular consensus-building around reform policies: ordinary people had very limited voice or influence over policy development and implementation. Policy-making was very top-down in approach and governments had made few attempts to consult civil society institutions on appropriate policy development. In some instances, notably in India, a very active NGO sector had emerged which had succeeded in pushing government to address certain key issues such as regulation. In both India and Thailand, a free and active media had helped to broaden out the debate on certain policy issues and had been instrumental in forcing government action on key issues (again, regulation was a prime example). However, these were notable exceptions to the general picture of small, closed, policy-making circles.

2.2   Capacity to implement new delivery structures

Internal aspects of capacity

All of the core country case studies had identified capacity problems relating to the number, skills and motivation of staff, although the nature and magnitude of these problems varied between countries. In Ghana, significant strides had been made in the development of a cadre of trained regional and district level public health managers, but it was observed that more trained accountants and finance officers were required.

In Zimbabwe there were perceived to be insufficient numbers of staff able to take on the jobs associated with the new roles of government, from revenue clerks at the facility level to managers at the provincial level. Often staff lacked the necessary skills and training; this ranged from lack of basic numeracy amongst staff responsible for book-keeping, to lack of more sophisticated skills such as financial management and negotiation. In addition, staff were viewed to be poorly motivated, particularly as a consequence of declining real wages, the civil service reform programme, and the consequent breakdown in labour relations. Expatriate technical advisers responsible for training a core group of skilled managers at the centre had observed that there was an absence of a managerial culture based on objective-setting and monitoring of performance. Managers were not accustomed to basing decisions upon analysis of information and did not give priority to collection or analysis of information.

In Sri Lanka, staff had possessed adequate basic administrative and management capacities so, for example, establishing contracts for straightforward services such as food purchasing could be managed. However, staff were poorly motivated to take on and perform well new roles such as those relating to regulation, and contracting out more complex services. Staff were disinclined to base decision-making upon information and had little incentive to do so.

There had appeared to be adequate skills to perform new government roles in India particularly at higher levels of the health system, and senior managers had often seemed to perform effectively. But for staff at lower levels, the incentives for good performance were weak, and low motivation to achieve organisational goals was widespread. Ineffective human resource management systems had played a large part in this problem. In addition to the highly centralised, rigid personnel management system in India, a parallel informal system also operated, on the basis of 'favours' and patronage. For example staff assigned to work in rural areas would vigorously lobby senior personnel in the Department for a transfer. The granting of such a transfer would then make them indebted to the grantor. The incentives which this informal system promoted were therefore likely to conflict with and potentially undermine the incentives which a performance-oriented personnel management system would promote.

In contrast to some of the core case study countries, the Thai bureaucracy had traditionally been viewed as highly competent, and indeed it appeared on the whole that the Thai government had experienced fewer internal capacity constraints in performing both old and new roles (perhaps with the exception of regulation) than governments elsewhere. Good basic administrative, management and planning skills and competencies were well established in the Thai bureaucracy. Until recently there had been a scarcity of higher- level analytical skills for complex tasks such as monitoring and evaluation, but training efforts during the late 1980s and early 1990s had helped to establish this capacity within the MOPH.

Problems of poor staff motivation observed in all four of the core countries were partially attributable to relatively low pay. In both the Sub-Saharan African countries, health worker pay had declined over time as a consequence of economic crisis. More generally, salaries for skilled health workers in the public sector were often considerably less than they could earn privately and in some instances (e.g. Zimbabwe and India until the recent pay review) public sector salaries were not considered adequate to live on. This created its own set of problems, particularly petty corruption and bribery. Bribery was reportedly problematic amongst officials working as inspectors in regulatory offices in India. Informal charges for health services were widespread in Ghana and India, and seemed to be becoming increasingly prevalent in Zimbabwe. Such informal charging may in the longer run undermine formal user-fee systems. More generally, health sector reform commonly requires health workers to invest their energies in learning new and complex tasks and acquiring new skills (Bennett and Franco 1999). Workers with low levels of motivation are most unlikely to be willing to make this investment.

The internal support systems which were most commonly identified as weak and contributing to government's incapacity to perform certain roles were financial systems and information systems (see Table 8.1). Weak financial systems were particularly important in undermining user fee reform in both Ghana and Zimbabwe. They also contributed to late payment of contractors in India. Absent or poor information systems were viewed as a barrier to reform in all core countries (see Table 8.2).

Part of the problem with information systems was that managers tended not to value information, particularly of certain types, and therefore gave such systems low priority. Information was used in a routine way for planning and budgeting, but most health planners and managers tended to focus upon health statistics and paid little attention to data (where it existed) on costs, efficiency and effectiveness. Information systems were highly centralised even in relatively decentralised contexts.

Budgetary and planning processes tended to be predictable and incremental rather than attempting to reorient the organisation in any

Table 8.2   The impact of weak information systems on specific reforms

Reform	Identified weakness in information system	Impact of weakness
Autonomous hospitals	Cost accounting systems poorly developed and returns generally late and incomplete	Difficult to move towards performance-based budgeting without first strengthening systems
User fees	Limited financial data available (e.g. revenues generated, exemptions given, spending profiles) Non-compliance with new financial information systems (Ghana)	Weakens monitoring of: collection mechanisms, effectiveness of exemptions, and appropriateness of spending decisions
Contracting out	Limited data on public sector costs or performance	Makes it difficult to evaluate wisdom of contracting out service
Regulation	Absence of complete database on private providers	No list to use for conducting inspections of private providers
	Inadequate systems for collecting information on case load in private sector	Difficult to compile complete picture of health service provision and hence to develop policies towards the private sector
	Inadequate records kept by private sector providers	Difficulty of proving or disproving cases of medical malpractice

substantial way. They were also very centralised in all of the countries examined. A commentator on Thailand observed that personnel, planning and budgeting systems did not encourage innovative thinking but were *'bureaucratic and concerned with procedures rather than strategy'* (Green 1997).

In the South Asian countries in particular, administrative systems were strong but over-bureaucratic and over-complex, discouraging strategic analysis and planning. While such centralised, bureaucratic systems may not create direct barriers to new forms of government (unlike inadequate financial or information systems), they do induce an organisational culture which is not conducive to the successful implementation of New Public Management approaches. For example, centralised planning systems are likely to emphasise adherence to centrally set goals and targets rather than local responsiveness to client-articulated needs.

While it was not a central focus of this study, other researchers have argued that too frequently donors have contributed to problems of weak capacity within Ministries of Health and other government agencies. Incompatible donor systems for planning and monitoring aid may divert limited government capacity away from reform planning and implementation to aid management (Walt et al. 1999). In the extreme situation *'more time and effort can be spent simply on handling donors than on developing the capacity to handle problems independently'* (Bikales 1997). Furthermore, despite the increasing emphasis amongst donors on capacity development (Morgan 1999), there is still a tendency for donors to establish their own individual enclaves for project implementation rather than building capacity in the system more broadly.

Weak coordination and communication between actors was a commonly perceived problem, and decentralisation policies which had been implemented without clear and explicit guidelines often further complicated coordination. In Sri Lanka with respect to regulation, and in Ghana with respect to autonomous hospitals, the central level had failed to set out clearly who should do what and this led to substantial confusion. Regulation often raised particularly acute problems of coordination, for a number of reasons: first, there was often, for historical reasons, a lack of trust between government and private sector actors; second, the objectives of such actors often differed substantially; and third, the sheer number of different actors involved in different aspects of regulation complicated coordination.

External factors affecting capacity

Many of the internal constraints discussed in the previous section were rooted not within the MOH but within the broader public sector institutional context (see Box 8.1).

Not only were the formal bureaucratic systems highly centralised, but the informal values, norms and conventions which constituted the management culture of these bureaucracies also tended to be centralised. Thus in some instances (such as APVVP – the autonomous hospital organisation in Andhra Pradesh), despite substantive formal reforms, the informal norms meant that the style of work changed only minimally. APVVP managed to make substantial improvements whilst a dynamic director was in place who was willing to disregard traditional management styles, but when other more traditional directors took over, it appeared that the organisation did not make full use of its autonomous status and managers deferred to officials within the state department of health (Chawla and George 1996).

Box 8.1   How overcentralised bureaucratic structures impede health sector reform

The case studies found numerous instances where state-wide bureaucratic regulations had impeded the progress of health sector reform. Specific examples included:

- price-fixing by the Ministry of Finance for certain types of contract (such as cleaning) in Thailand;
- reversion of user fee revenues to the central treasury in Zimbabwe (until 1996 reforms);
- centralised (and rather opaque) tendering procedures in Ghana in which MOH representatives had very limited involvement;
- inability to fire public sector employees in Tamil Nadu which meant that contracting-out of existing services (such as the proposed laundry contract) was not cost-effective.

Centralised personnel systems and financial systems in particular were singled out for criticism. Personnel regulations set by civil service commissions left local level managers with very little control over the key input to health services: staffing. Common problems associated with such systems were: over-staffing, inability to fire staff (even for appalling performance), a lack of relationship between performance and reward, and frequently relatively high pay for unskilled staff compared to the private sector. These problems permeated not only traditional delivery structures but prevented many of the reforms from operating effectively.

Ministries of Finance were commonly criticised for being fixed in a 'policing' mode rather than an enabling mode. Centralised financial systems emphasised control rather than producing relevant financial information for managers. Consequently there was limited financial or cost data available at the local level and no culture of using such information for decision-making.

A variety of aspects of the political, economic and social environment were seen to impede government's capacity to implement new delivery structures. Several problems associated with 'political interference' were identified; however, many of these related to the design of the reform agenda rather than the operation of reformed institutions. One example

where political considerations clearly affected the successful implementation of reforms was the user-fee programme in Ghana. Whilst it would
have been desirable to increase fees routinely in line with inflation, the
political sensitivity of this decision meant that it was necessary for
parliament to pass a new regulation each time fees needed to be increased.
This understandably prevented timely increases in fees.

Problems associated with implementing reform at a time of economic
crisis have already been discussed. The other element of the economic
environment which the case studies addressed was the extent of private
sector development. For contracting out of services, the level of private
sector development was clearly a very pertinent issue as it affected the
number of possible contractors and hence the degree of competition in
the local market. It was a much greater binding constraint in the African
than South Asian context. The level of private sector development also
had a less direct, but more pervasive effect. A limited formal private sector
appeared disadvantageous in terms of lack of exposure of public sector
managers to new management techniques. In countries with a substantial
private sector such as India, techniques and tools such as quality
improvement, contracting out, and performance-related pay were likely
to be much more widely understood and discussed than in countries
where there was a very limited private sector. Furthermore government
might be able to recruit experienced private sector managers more easily
(albeit at a cost) than in countries without a substantial private sector. In
industrialised countries, New Public Management has sought to import
private sector management techniques into the public sector: in
developing countries those management techniques are often not very
well rooted even in the private sector.

Issues of corruption were discussed particularly in the Indian case study
but there was suggestive evidence that they were also a problem
elsewhere. While the controls inherent in bureaucratic systems are
designed to curtail corrupt activities by civil servants, corruption is likely
to thrive in over-centralised, rule-bound, bureaucratic systems where
bribery and extortion appear simpler paths than following the letter of the
law (Klitgaard 1991). Corruption may be further encouraged by very low
government salaries. It poses a number of constraints upon the effective
implementation of new forms of service delivery:

- corruption at lower levels of government, and the difficulty of
  monitoring resource use at lower levels, was a reason very frequently
  cited by central government officials for caution in pursuing
  decentralisation policies;

- the personal and political benefits which may accrue from control over large central contracts is probably an important (though infrequently cited) reason for central level opposition to the devolution of budgets;
- financial systems for monitoring the collection of user fees and revenue use may need to be particularly strong and closely monitored when corruption is an issue;
- contracting in a corrupt context may mean that the contract is not awarded to the most efficient supplier;
- problems of corruption may prevent regulatory processes from being carried out properly (for example, providers may bribe inspectors rather than meet set standards), and divert subsidies and other enabling measures away from their intended beneficiaries, so that neither of these types of measures achieve their intended effect.

Problems related to corruption pervade traditional modes of government as well as impede new forms of government, and there are ways in which these new forms can be structured so as at least to deter corrupt activities: for example, complete transparency about tendering processes and selection of successful tenders should help avoid corrupt awarding of contracts. However, in an environment where corruption is pervasive, implementing such discrete reforms may be of limited effectiveness.

In India, as a direct consequence of widespread corruption, there was an acute mistrust of government by the general population. This had resulted in substantial difficulties in implementing certain policies. For example, the new regulatory statute in Tamil Nadu was seen by many providers as a ruse to enable corrupt government officials to add to their income, and as a consequence many private sector actors were strongly opposed to the legislation and planned to resist registration.

3. Key issues for capacity building in health sector reform

While countries and different reform policies faced diverse sets of capacity constraints, a number of key issues for capacity building for health sector reform emerge from the above analysis:

- *Recognising the importance of, and developing skills to manage, the transition process* – including development of clear policy frameworks, phasing of reforms, communication of reforms and garnering commitment to reforms, development of rational and realistic implementation plans.

- *Ensuring adequate basic capacities* – there has been severe decay in government performance of basic routine administrative functions in countries which have experienced acute economic crisis. In such contexts, rebuilding basic government roles must be given priority.
- *Addressing organisational culture* – it takes a long time for people to absorb and come to terms with reforms which are designed to change the very culture of the work place. In all countries studied (including Thailand) the organisational culture was based upon hierarchy, command and duty, favours and patronage; consequently there was little incentive for staff to innovate. Capacity building needs to pay attention not only to the more tangible aspects of an organisation but also to the organisational culture.
- *Coping with external constraints* – while traditional approaches to capacity building have tended to focus upon the development of skills and systems, it seems that frequently binding capacity constraints lie outside of the ministry of health (or other responsible organisation). In particular, over-centralised bureaucracy-wide regulations, entrenched corruption and the instability associated with frequent political change and inconsistent direction from the political level may inhibit effective reform regardless of the level of internal capacity.
- *Phasing reforms* – none of the study countries had paid much conscious attention to the question of how best to phase specific reform programmes (or indeed the overall structure of reform programmes); however, the capacity constraints described here imply that reforms need to be carefully planned and phased so as to build upon available capacity while gradually expanding capacity to undertake new tasks.

Each of these aspects of capacity building is addressed in more detail below.

3.1   Transition capacity

While there are many different ways in which to understand the policy process, Walt (1994) has argued that in general, decisions of 'high politics' or decisions regarding systemic issues are made by relatively small policy elites whereas more micro policies tend to show the influence of a broader range of policy and civil society groupings. In the case studies examined here, a substantial amount of decision-making about the scope and direction of reform seems to have rested in the hands of a very small policy elite: namely senior national technocrats and external policy advisors. This situation led to a number of adverse consequences.

First, implementation of reforms suffered due to lack of ownership of reform programmes on the part of key stakeholders such as politicians, health workers and health service users. New Public Management-type reforms are perhaps particularly prone to such problems. As Hirschmann observed:

> the very people who were most threatened by these policy reforms were the ones who were expected to carry them out; government agencies and personnel were expected to co-operate in diminishing or dismantling their own power. (Hirschmann 1993)

Donors may exacerbate these problems: other analysts have high-lighted the fact that external consultants provided by donors tend to be selected for their technical expertise rather than their ability to facilitate a process of reform (Wight 1997). Consequently, little attempt is made to involve other stakeholders and discussion of reforms tends to take place in a highly technical language which may not be accessible to those outside the policy elite.

Second, while reform proposals may have been technically sound they were not always politically feasible. The technocratic perspective of many donors and external consultants probably contributed to this problem.

Third, the almost complete exclusion of implementers from policy circles had implications not only for the ownership of reforms but also for reform designs. This was particularly evident in the Sub-Saharan African countries, where a common understanding amongst the policy elite about the direction of the reform programme could result in relatively sophisticated programmes and plans which masked real difficulties in implementation.

The problems which occur when there is lack of local ownership of aid projects have long been recognised, and many donors have taken measures to promote greater local ownership of their projects (Wight 1997). However, the case studies conducted here suggest that problems persist, especially in the Sub-Saharan African countries, and that these problems are particularly critical when it is a programme of policy reform which lacks ownership rather than one particular development project.

Donor dominance of reform programmes is exacerbated by weak routine government planning systems which have little if any strategic content.[1] Hence more radical realignment of policies tends to be donor-led. Working to strengthen and make annual and other routine planning processes more strategic is therefore an important step in establishing stronger local ownership of reform programmes.

In addition, donors and policy-makers alike need to ensure that there is acceptance of and commitment to reforms amongst a broader group of stakeholders and that practical implementation perspectives are brought in at the early stages of policy formulation. For a major reform initiative, political and stakeholder analyses may help reformers understand the agenda of key interest groups. Ensuring that reforms are in alignment with political goals is a crucial step in securing political support. Alliances between reform-oriented actors must be built and barriers to change negotiated, if contentious policy initiatives are to have any chance of adoption and implementation.

Once the broad strategy of reforms has been agreed upon, communicating this vision to others and building consensus and support around the vision is important, but was largely ignored in the case study countries. While Ministries of Health may be accustomed to the social marketing of family planning supplies, the notion of needing to market a programme of reforms is still in its infancy. Only in Thailand was the MOPH beginning to think about its role in information provision with respect to health system organisation and reform. Strengthening information, education and communication capacities within Ministries of Health to perform such a function (or alternatively, getting ministries to recognise the importance of IEC in policy reform and to contract for such services) is a relatively straightforward step which should be undertaken.

Finally, all leaders of reform processes need to acknowledge that even once a clear policy statement and commitment to reform amongst key stakeholders exists, much work in terms of defining implementation plans remains to be done prior to implementation. In Sub-Saharan African countries at least, an absolute lack of capacity within government hindered the successful completion of this critical step. While consultants can help with the process of translating policies into operational plans, operational details often imbue policies with a very particular flavour and for local ownership to be maintained, this task cannot be handed over wholesale to external consultants. A final lesson, then, is the need to be less ambitious in reform programmes: to try to identify those reforms which may potentially unlock self-sustaining reform programmes, and to try to do these discrete reforms well, rather than taking on an over-ambitious agenda.

3.2   Strengthening basic capacities

Traditional approaches to capacity building include training (both on-the-job and special training courses), technical assistance, development of guidelines and manuals, and study tours to see how systems operate elsewhere. Such approaches were quite prevalent in the study countries. For example, the Ghanaian authorities had used training workshops to develop user-fee management capacity, and had sent a number of more senior staff overseas for training in public health as part of the capacity building efforts for decentralisation. Similarly in Zimbabwe, external donors had provided technical assistance to help develop guidelines for contracting out non-clinical services, and expatriate personnel had also contributed to the development of financial management systems and skills in preparation for decentralisation.

These approaches are all still relevant to the new roles of government. Skills such as those in financial management and analysis, legal drafting and economics are probably best acquired through formal training. However, many of the critical skills required to operationalise effectively the new reforms cannot easily be taught through formal training, but are instead skills learnt through experience, trial and error (Paul 1995). Reform programmes need to build opportunities for individuals to assess experience to date and learn from their own (or others') mistakes. Technical assistance had seemed to play a critical role on occasion in both Ghana and Zimbabwe in helping local personnel to transform new policies into practical approaches, sometimes including development of guidelines and manuals.

However, whilst traditional approaches to capacity building were still clearly of relevance, there was sometimes a danger that they received excessive attention whilst other capacity issues (such as external constraints, lack of consensus around the reforms, or poor coordination between actors) were more binding but were addressed to only a limited extent.

3.3   Addressing organisational culture

Organisational culture can be defined as *'a shared set of norms and behavioral expectations characterizing a corporate identity'* (Grindle 1997). Few government organisations in developing countries have made a conscious effort to develop a particular organisational culture;[2] instead the organisational culture evolves from the pervading organisational structures, systems, personnel and leadership and their interaction with broader societal culture (such as the importance given to hierarchy, or collective versus individualistic behaviour).

Although organisational cultures are not static and are likely to change over time as the organisation itself evolves, they tend to be very deeply embedded. It is unlikely, therefore, that reform of the structure of the organisation alone will bring about rapid change in organisational culture (Morgan 1986). Hence it seems essential to consider the role played by organisational culture if reforms are to take root and be effective. The case studies found numerous examples where change had occurred in the outward form of an organisation or training had taken place, but it seemed that attitudes and values of the people within the organisation had not changed accordingly and hence there had been very little impact. Other analysts in the health sector have highlighted the same problem:

> The system becomes resistant to change that does not serve the implicit values in use: and, as long as these values are not openly acknowledged their effects cannot be discussed or predicted. If planning and management efforts continue to ignore the presence of these values in use within the organisation, they will continue to fail to create change. (Aitken 1994)

Culture within an organisation is critically dependent upon the human resource management systems which govern recruitment and promotions as these determine the character of individuals within the organisation and who become 'formal' leaders or supervisors. Previous sections have already highlighted the considerable array of problems associated with the centralised human resource management systems existing in all of the case study countries. Without control over these systems, Ministries of Health are likely to find it extremely difficult to change organisational culture. For example, the Ghana case study had noted that:

> The persistence of inflexible, cumbersome and highly centralised personnel management procedures encourages nepotism and dis-courages risk taking. (Smithson, Asamoa-Baah and Mills 1995)

Charismatic or transformational leadership is another element which may succeed in changing organisational culture. None of the case studies examined as part of this research had identified this as a significant influence in the reform programmes, although many respondents in India had acknowledged the importance of credible leadership in increasing the public's trust in an organisation. In countries where more radical health sector reform programmes have been pursued, transforma-tional leaders appear to have played an important role in terms not only of specific structural reforms but also of creating a stronger sense of calling and organisational mission amongst those working in the health sector. Studies of the health sector reform processes in both South Africa and

Zambia (which have pursued relatively radical reforms) identified the critical importance of strong political leadership in reform processes (Daura et al. 1999, CHP and HEU 1999). Another study of reform in Sub-Saharan Africa identified Health Ministers as an important source of leadership for reform (UNICEF 1998). Strong leadership has also been identified as a critical factor in the development of local government capacity, particularly in terms of promoting motivation amongst staff:

> Leadership was a sine qua non in the launching, and figured importantly in the sustaining, of capacity building... This leadership function has a double facet. First reforming the municipal administration into a more effective and customer oriented institution involves a leadership role internal to the organisation. Second, achieving trust, mobilising community resources and sustaining those reform efforts involve a leadership role external to the organisation. (Fiszbein 1997)

From this discussion, it should be clear that while generating change in organisational culture may be key to the effective implementation of reforms, it is likely to be a very complex task and progress will most likely be limited by the close links between organisational culture and broader societal culture. Without strong political leadership, transforming organisational culture will be particularly difficult. An alternative approach, worthy of more consideration, is to assess how reform programmes can be reconfigured to take account better of existing organisational culture.

In a couple of the countries studied (India and Ghana),[3] there were efforts to bypass broader bureaucratic constraints and establish new autonomous organisations which might develop an organisational culture untainted by that of the broader public sector. Such organisations would not be bound by public service regulations and hence managers would have far greater flexibility in how they hired and rewarded staff. Grindle (1997) concluded that such 'elite' units (or enclave agencies) outside the main government bureaucracy frequently exhibit higher levels of performance. She attributed this partly to a much stronger performance orientation within such units, combined with independent and meritocratic recruitment. The evidence, however, is not entirely clear: while such agencies may be successful in achieving high-priority tasks, they may create resentment in other parts of the civil service, be only weakly accountable, and delay more fundamental reform of the bureaucratic constraints which prevent effective government performance (World Bank 1997). In India it was evident that the autonomous organisations created often had relatively weak channels of accountability and did not form part of a broader strategy to reform the government sector.

3.4   Coping with external constraints

Analysts have observed that governments and donor agencies frequently pay too little attention to the external environment which may form the critically binding constraint on implementation of policies (Brinkerhoff 1994). This is perhaps understandable: tackling a wide range of external constraints is likely to appear an intimidating and most likely unrewarding task. However, the study findings presented here have indicated that the external environment frequently prevents or delays reforms, and consequently suggest that policy-makers and advisers need to find better ways to cope with these external constraints.

It is useful to distinguish between two types of constraint external to the Ministry of Health: first, those constraints rooted in the broader public sector institutional context; and second, constraints stemming from the political, economic and social context. While the Ministry of Health alone may be able to do little to lift the first set of constraints, they are none the less likely to be more tractable than the second set. Health sector agencies can at least lobby central ministries for changes in regulations which are found to be particularly constraining, or pilot schemes can sometimes be exempted from the usual regulations and used to demonstrate the benefits of alternative approaches. A further option, as discussed above, is the establishment of elite or enclave agencies outside standard civil service regulations. None the less, the links between health sector reform and broader public sector institutional reform are strong and do constrain the scope for radical change in the health sector alone.

Problems stemming from the political, economic and social context are likely to be considerably harder to relieve. The main types of issues for health sector reform, identified above, were:

- political 'interference' in policy making and implementation;
- the impact of economic crisis on policy implementation;
- the level of private sector development;
- corruption.

None of these problems is likely to be tractable to health sector-specific approaches. Consequently health policy-makers need to find ways to work round them. It may be possible to compensate internally for some environmental constraints through careful reform design. For example, some of the problems associated with corruption may be alleviated by establishing transparent tendering procedures. Political interference in health sector management may potentially be reduced by careful definition of those decisions where political interference is legitimate and those where managers are allowed freedom of choice. Strengthening channels of downward accountability to communities may also make it harder for politicians to intervene. Limited private sector development may not be an insurmountable barrier to contracting out certain services if the possibility exists of organising bids by public sector work units. Although some negative impact on reform programmes stemming from economic crisis probably cannot be prevented, realistic implementation plans which allow for limited resource availability may minimise it.

In some instances, constraints in the political, economic and social context will mean that certain reforms are neither feasible nor desirable. For example, Schick argues that the development of adequate market institutions is a logical precursor to the strengthening of public sector management using a contracts-based approach (Schick 1998). It is possible to identify other instances where external constraints, such as political turbulence, crisis in government legitimacy or severe economic recession substantially curtail the potential menu of reform policies available to government.

More generally, health sector reform is often part of a broader agenda of social reform. While health sector reform may have its own specific goals (such as increasing access to care or improving quality of care), many of the mechanisms through which government is striving to achieve these goals have broader social implications. As the former Minister of Health in Zambia noted:

> The struggle over quality health care for our people is at once a struggle over political rule and about democratic empowerment. (Kalumba 1997)

Given the intimate linkages between health sector reform and broader social, economic and political development processes, it is probably inappropriate that these two strands of development become too out of step with each other.

3.5 Phasing reforms

Several analysts have pointed out that reforms are not 'all or nothing' events, but can be (and indeed in reality generally are) progressive, incremental processes. For example:

New Public Management is not just an organisational reform but a long term learning process within public administration. The time dimension is often underestimated by reformers. (Klages and Loffler 1998)

And in considering the relevance of the use of formalised contracts in public sector reform programmes, Schick notes that:

significant progress can be made through a logical sequence of steps that diminish the scope of informality while building managerial capacity, confidence and experience. (Schick 1998)

Perhaps one of the most constructive lessons from the foregoing analysis concerns the importance of careful phasing of reform programmes. A number of criteria need to be taken into account:

- *Existing health system* – different countries have different starting points in terms of the existing design of the health system and the previous history of reform. While analysts have repeatedly asserted that there is no standard reform package, and indeed in an ideal world there should not be, analysis of the case studies presented here suggests that in reality the prescription being offered across countries does have very similar elements. Country-specific analysis needs to identify which of the package of policies commonly associated with New Public Management and health sector reform is most relevant to, and of highest priority in, the context under consideration.
- *Existing capacity* – different countries also have different institutional endowments or capacities. Capacity strengths and weaknesses should be identified and the reform programme should build upon the strengths, whether this be strong financial management or a history of community participation. Perhaps most critically, every step should be taken to ensure that existing capacities are not destroyed during a transition process.
- *Political realities* – political support for reforms may be difficult to secure over a sufficiently long period to see benefits reaped from the entire reform programme. There are considerable advantages to reform programmes which deliver some benefits early on to key stakeholders, thus helping maintain commitment to reforms.
- *Breaking reform into bite-size chunks* – all four of the tracer reforms considered in this book could be broken down into smaller components which build upon each other. For example, prior to granting full autonomy to a health provider, steps could first be taken to strengthen

financial management systems within the organisation and then resource allocation changed to a system of global budgets which allows the organisation far greater flexibility in resource management. Similarly, implementation of user fees need not be pursued system-wide: as experience in Kenya showed (Collins et al. 1996), there may be much to recommend a process of implementing fees first at higher-level referral hospitals then working slowly down the health system, continually expanding financial management capacity as the reform is implemented. In contracting for health care, it makes good sense to start with certain non-clinical services which can be more easily specified in advance and monitored, prior to expanding contracting to more complex services (Bennett and Mills 1998).

- *Technical complexity of reforms* – some reforms are innately more complex than others and likely to require considerably greater capacity to implement successfully. For example, of the reforms considered in this book, effective regulation of private providers would seem inherently more difficult to design and implement well than a good user-fee policy.

- *Interrelationship amongst different reform elements* – some types of reform may be mutually supportive. For example, it is fairly commonly accepted that quality improvements need to be made at the same time (or prior to) the introduction of user fees. However, our understanding of the interrelationship amongst other aspects of reform programmes is more limited: for example, is it logical to introduce user fees prior to giving hospitals autonomy or decentralising services? Furthermore, a particular type of capacity may support more than one reform: for example, strengthened financial management may support both stronger autonomy and greater revenue collection; such complementarities would also affect appropriate timing.

To date, virtually no research into the appropriate phasing of health sector reform programmes has been undertaken: this issue requires further research and analysis.

4. Towards a strategy for capacity building

Bearing in mind the complexity of the concept of capacity and its context-specific nature, this section pulls together the lessons emerging from the analyses in this and previous chapters with findings from other studies of capacity, in order to outline a preliminary strategy for capacity building for health sector reform programmes. Figure 8.1 provides an overview of

194

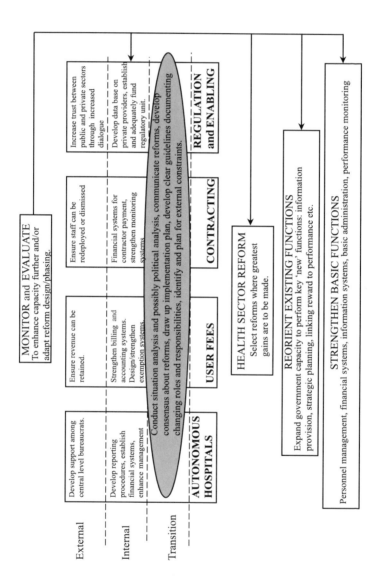

Figure 8.1 Capacity building for health sector reform

the elements of this strategy. The most fundamental elements of capacity building for health sector reform are indicated at the base of the figure. Further up the figure, more task-specific forms of capacity building are illustrated for the four tracer reforms considered in the study.

A substantial amount has been written about capacity building and institutional development. From this body of work has emerged some general principles and some quite detailed recommendations for how to proceed with capacity building strategies.[4] While very little of this work is health sector-specific, many of the conclusions and recommendations are in line with the findings of this study. The primary conclusions from this literature, in terms of general principles for capacity building, are as follows:

- capacity building is by nature incremental and slow; consequently, actors involved in capacity building need to accept the relatively long time-frame for significant results to be achieved;
- different capacity constraints are evident in different contexts and for different types of functions or roles; hence there is no blueprint for resolving problems of capacity: interventions to strengthen capacity need to be rooted in a situation-specific analysis of the key constraints;
- similarly, reform programmes should be designed to take into account existing capacity; capacity is a resource or an institutional endowment, and reform programmes need to work out how best they can make use of this resource;
- reform programmes should be designed so as to start with those changes which can be relatively easily implemented given existing capacity. Reforms which require capacities currently not present in the system should, if possible, be left until later stages of the reform programme. Reforms which are likely to be blocked by aspects of the external environment over which reformers have little control should be delayed or avoided altogether.

Though capacity building may at first appear to be an intimidating task, it is possible to create virtuous cycles. There is evidence to suggest that efficient organisations are better able to attract high-quality staff and motivate those staff to high levels of performance (Fiszbein 1997, Tendler 1997). Even relatively small steps in capacity building may lead to higher, sustainable outcomes.

There was considerable variation in performance of basic functions across the study countries. While on the whole, basic administrative functions and financial and information systems operated effectively in Sri Lanka and Thailand, in the other countries there were problems with some basic bureaucratic functions. Inadequate capacity to perform such basic functions adversely affects both traditional modes of government and 'new' service arrangements, and where such problems occur, capacity building needs to start at this level. The three key sets of systems which were commonly found to be weak and hence formed obstacles to effective health sector reforms were personnel management systems, financial systems and information systems. Strengthening of each of these systems will contribute towards the capacity necessary to implement reform policies. For example, autonomous hospitals require financial systems to enable them to account for funds received; user fees require strong financial systems to help health workers manage revenues and expenditures; and in order to be able to contract effectively, governments need to be able to pay contractors on time.

Some functions such as information provision have traditionally been viewed as functions of government, but government has carried them out only to a limited degree. Other functions such as planning and budgeting have been assiduously performed, but as largely bureaucratic processes with little evident impact upon improving equity, efficiency or effectiveness. Similarly, governments have always been responsible for remunerating public sector health workers and distributing budgets between health facilities, but in general this task has been done with little regard for performance. Reorienting the way in which these tasks are managed will help establish the necessary prerequisites for NPM-type reforms, but may also strengthen government performance of traditional forms of service delivery. Many of these functions can be gradually reoriented; they do not require sweeping reforms. For example, programme budgeting can be gradually introduced at different levels of the health system. Linking staff reward to performance may start not with basic salaries but by making a clearer link between performance and certain perquisites or access to training. Gradual reorientation of these existing functions will begin to change the organisational culture of the MOH.

The following chapter addresses directly the question of the wisdom of adopting NPM-type reforms; however, from the perspective of capacity, it is clear that many governments have experienced considerable problems in implementing comprehensive reform programmes. Reformers need to be selective: they should identify those policies and changes which are both most feasible and are likely to yield the most benefits. Organisational culture should be taken into account: certain reforms (for example, decentralisation) may have a widespread impact on the way in which health workers approach their job. Reforms such as this can be a key to more broad-based change throughout the health system.

Whatever the reforms agreed upon, there are a number of basic steps necessary for the transition process. To start with, a situation analysis should be conducted so that there is clarity over current arrangements, existing capacities and the system-level changes that will need to be made to introduce the proposed reform. For major reform initiatives, a political or stakeholder analysis should also be undertaken so that potential obstacles to reform can be identified and negotiated. The reform needs to be communicated, both so that implementers are completely clear about the purpose and content of reform and in order to build support for reforms. The target audience for this information and the content of the message will differ depending on the reform. For example, for autonomous hospitals, broadcasting a message to both health workers and the public that autonomy is not a first step towards privatisation may be an important element of gaining support and consensus about the reform. Informing people of the problems found amongst private health providers may help generate a demand for regulation amongst the general public. Other necessary steps in building transition capacity include drawing up realistic implementation plans, developing clear guidelines which document changing roles and responsibilities for the new service delivery arrangements, and identifying and planning for external constraints.

As capacity is task-specific, different reforms will require capacity building efforts to focus on different areas. Priorities for internal and external capacity building for each of the four reforms considered in this book were illustrated in Figure 8.1. They include:

- *for autonomous hospitals:* developing reporting procedures between the hospital and the MOH, enhancing hospital management and establishing appropriate internal financial systems, as well as working with central level bureaucrats to reduce their opposition to such a form of decentralisation;
- *for user fees:* strengthening billing and accounting systems, and designing or strengthening exemption mechanisms, as well as ensuring that fee revenues can be retained at an appropriate level within the health care system;
- *for contracting out:* strengthening financial systems for contractor payment and monitoring systems, as well as ensuring that the staff currently performing the service to be contracted can be redeployed or removed;
- *for regulation and enabling:* developing and maintaining a database on private health care providers; establishing and adequately funding a

regulatory unit as well as working to increase trust between public and private sectors through increased dialogue.

Finally, the dynamic dimension of capacity is critical. Enabling policy-makers and implementers to learn from the reforms implemented is essential. Furthermore, even in the best-planned reform programme there are likely to be continuous amendments and adjustments: health workers and health systems must be prepared for continuing adaptation. Ongoing monitoring and evaluation should be conducted with the participation of the implementers. Lessons emerging can be fed back to implementers and systems adapted accordingly so as to strengthen capacity further.

5.   Conclusions

This chapter has amplified the analytical framework used to assess capacity and reviewed the multiple capacity problems identified in the case-studies. Key capacity constraints were found to be:

- lack of consensus and/or lack of understanding of reforms, meaning that although reforms were officially adopted, implementation never properly started;
- hurried implementation of reforms due to pressures external to Ministries of Health, resulting in inadequate planning for reform and unrealistic time-frames for implementation;
- shortages of certain specialised skills (e.g. contract design and negotiation) preventing implementation;
- staff poorly motivated to invest personal energies in learning new skills and tasks for reform;
- weak financial, information and personnel management systems;
- public sector rules and regulations which impeded specific reforms within the health sector and contributed towards an organisational culture which emphasised process (particularly following rules) over achieving good outcomes.

A number of capacity building strategies were identified to help address these problems. In addition it was argued that reform programmes need to be phased so as to reflect and build upon existing capacities.

Health sector reform commonly implies new and more complex roles for government. For government to be able to fulfil these new roles effectively, it is often necessary not only to strengthen systems and enhance health workers' skills but also to change the organisational culture prevailing within the public sector. While the internal capacity problems summarised in this chapter have formed significant constraints in the case study countries to successful reform implementation, on their own they probably do not constitute a sufficient reason for not implementing reforms. Indeed, many of the capacity problems analysed here are also problematic under traditional forms of service delivery. With well-planned efforts to enhance internal capacity and carefully phased reforms, it may be possible, over time, to address many of the constraints identified here. External constraints – such as rigid public sector-wide regulations, the absolute lack of resources in countries facing economic crisis, widespread corruption and political interference – are harder to address and may jeopardise the reform programme.

These conclusions on capacity building leave unanswered the question of whether the potential gains to be made from implementing an NPM-influenced health sector reform agenda outweigh the likely costs in terms of investments necessary to enhance capacity. Chapter 9 turns to the fundamental question of the relevance and appropriateness of NPM-type reforms to the health sectors of developing countries.

9
Reforming Health Sector Reform

1.   Capacity to do what?

The previous chapter addressed both the capacity problems faced by those case study countries that had considered or introduced specific reforms, and how capacity might best be increased. It left largely unaddressed the fundamental question of the relevance of these reform measures to particular countries, and indeed the relevance of what is widely perceived to be an international health sector reform agenda based on NPM principles. While the evidence that capacity constraints are a severe barrier to the implementation of reforms provides a *prima facie* case for questioning those reforms, it is also important to address directly the relevance of reforms.

This final chapter, therefore, questions the overall reform agenda, and the value of the specific reforms that are the focus of this book, as well as drawing conclusions on the difficulties of implementing health sector reform policies. The initial sections provide a summary and drawing together of the content of earlier chapters, giving an overview of the extent of reform in the case study countries, and of the performance of governments overall as well as in relation to the specific policies examined. The chapter then goes on to question the relevance of NPM and its associated policies to country circumstances. Finally, the chapter concludes by identifying the need for a new approach to reform; one more deeply rooted in and sensitive to the institutional characteristics of individual countries.

2.   The international health sector reform agenda and its adoption in the countries

Chapter 1 referred to the current wave of interest in changing policies, practices and management systems within the health sector, and identified a number of elements of what has become known as 'health sector reform'. There has been considerable questioning of whether it makes any sense to refer to an international health sector reform agenda (Marmor 1997), and it is true that at the country level, the components of reform can vary greatly. However, at the level of policy rhetoric, there is a surprising consistency in the pronouncements. Mackintosh has commented that:

> The conception of social policy as being the professional and/or hierarchical provision of welfare services is being actively replaced by a different image: that of provision by commercial and public interest bodies, with the state playing a regulatory, purchasing and residual provider role. (Mackintosh 1995)

The World Bank, in the much quoted *World Development Report* of 1993, emphasised improving the quality and efficiency of government services through decentralisation and performance-related incentives, and greater diversity and competition in the supply of health services, including competition between public and private providers (World Bank 1993).

The OECD, in its 1992 review of the reform of health care in seven OECD countries, identified signs of convergence on an approach to the financing and organisation of health care where funding is obtained from taxation or compulsory social insurance contributions, the financial intermediaries are public or quasi-public bodies, and they have contractual relationships with providers whether public or private: in other words, there is a separation between the funding organisations and providers in contrast to the traditional integrated approach of many publicly funded health systems (OECD 1992).

The agenda of the Inter-American Development Bank has some similar themes:

> Public finance and regulation, provider autonomy and consumer empowerment are the cornerstones of improved functioning...Public sources are better allocated according to outcomes and with increased autonomy by providers... Equity can be improved when access to services is guaranteed by the public funding that individuals bring with them to the ... clinic, rather than by proximity to a centrally planned facility. Consumer decision making powers can be strengthened with greater information regarding the quality of diverse providers, with greater voice in the functioning of purchasing agencies and providers and with greater options for choosing amongst numerous providers. (Inter-American Development Bank 1996)

The main components of this international health sector reform agenda, as argued in Chapter 1, are closely associated with NPM themes. They can be categorised within the framework of the key functions of a health system: regulation and enabling; financing; purchasing; and providing. Table 9.1 summarises the main areas of health sector reform within each of these. It also associates with them NPM rationales, and where the reforms were adopted or under consideration in the case study countries, identifies the main rationale for adopting these policies at country level.

Four key points emerge from this table.

First, adoption of NPM-type policies in a comprehensive reform agenda was very limited except in the two African countries: Ghana and Zimbabwe. Thailand had certain policies in place which had greatly encouraged the growth of the private sector, but with respect to the services under the control of the MOH, had shown little enthusiasm for NPM-type policies.

Second, even where countries had adopted NPM-type polices, their reasons for doing so often differed from the NPM rationale. This was particularly the case with respect to user fees, where the main concern was to raise revenue rather than to improve efficiency or empower consumers; and changing relationships with the private sector, where prime concerns were strengthened regulation to protect consumers and control dangerous and unethical behaviours, rather than active enabling.

Third, none of the countries had sought to implement a wide-ranging health sector reform agenda. In industrialised countries, and particularly in the UK and New Zealand, the package of reforms implemented (e.g. purchaser/provider splits; contracts; hospital autonomy) has been linked and mutually reinforcing. The one case study country that had a wide-ranging plan, Zimbabwe, had made little progress in translating it into reality. Although evidence is therefore lacking on issues associated with implementing a broad reform agenda, the fact that countries had had great difficulty in implementing even a very limited set of specific reforms casts doubt on the feasibility of a broader agenda.

Fourth, reforms in all countries were focused on restructuring and strengthening the public sector, for example, through decentralisation of health service management and restructuring Ministries of Health, rather than fundamentally changing the public sector's role in the overall health system. The broad structure of health services as between public and private sectors had remained largely unaffected by reform policy in the four core case study countries, albeit in Thailand the access to the private sector permitted by the introduction of compulsory insurance and expansion of medical benefit schemes had promoted its growth.

Table 9.1 The main areas of health sector reform, their NPM rationale and their adoption in reform agendas of case study countries

Key functions of health systems and main areas of health sector reform	NPM rationale	Whether part of case study country reform agenda, and rationale
Enabling Liberalising laws on private health sector and introducing incentives for expansion	To encourage pluralism in provision, consumer choice, and efficiency-enhancing competition	Liberal policies already present. Enabling to limited extent except Thailand, where aim to expand marketz
Regulation Revising regulatory structure	Not emphasised; greater emphasis on incentives rather than control	Yes – all countries, to protect consumers and ensure minimum quality standards
Financing • User fees • Community financing, including community-based insurance • Social health insurance (also in	To reduce need for tax funding To encourage money to follow patients; to increase accountability of providers to clients	In Ghana and Zimbabwe • User fees: to raise revenue for cash-starved health services • Social health insurance Thailand): to increase funding and allow tax funds to go to poorer groups
Purchasing • Creation of purchasing agencies and management agreements with providers • Introduction of competitive contractual relationships • Reforming payment systems	To ensure that interests of providers do not drive decisions on resource allocation To encourage competition between providers in order to increase efficiency and responsiveness to purchasers and users	• Purchaser/provider split: only in Zimbabwe and Ghana, to strengthen management control • Contracts: to limited extent in these countries and Thailand, mainly for non-clinical services • Reformed payment systems: in Thailand, to keep costs down and maintain quality

Table 9.1 (*continued*)

Key functions of health systems and main areas of health sector reform	NPM rationale	Whether part of case study country reform agenda, and rationale
Provision • Decentralisation of health service management • Increased autonomy to public hospitals • Improved accountability to service users and population	To give managers greater responsibility; allow consumers to have greater 'voice' in management	• All countries: some decentralisation of overall management to districts; Ghana: creation of an executive agency • Hospital autonomy: policy for teaching hospitals in Ghana/Zimbabwe; Thailand: policy for MOH hospitals under discussion • All countries: little attention to giving users a voice

3.   The need for reform

Can the very limited implementation of an NPM-influenced reform agenda be explained by generally adequate performance of traditional arrangements in the health sector? Overall, as Chapter 2 made clear, the case study countries demonstrated many of the problems which NPM reforms are designed to address.

The study countries represented differing degrees of effectiveness of government's performance of its traditional roles (and to some degree were selected because of this). Sri Lanka is widely regarded as a success with respect to the performance of its health sector,[1] and had very impressive health status outcomes for a country at its level of development. In contrast, much of India[2] had very poor health status outcomes for its level of income, with health services having had little evident impact on outcomes such as child survival (World Bank 1998).

In Sub-Saharan Africa, post-Independence Zimbabwe was recognised as a success story: significant improvements were made in health status through redressing inequalities in the sector and expanding coverage with basic services. However, it was not possible to sustain this record (UNICEF 1994). The health sector in Ghana had been subject to pressures for expansion since Independence. As a consequence, the government sector was very large, to the point of being overextended. Health status indicators were typical of Sub-Saharan Africa (or slightly worse).

The catalogue of problems with government performance was strikingly similar across countries almost regardless of health status outcomes. In India, poor staff motivation and poor drug supplies combined with dilapidated government infrastructure were significant problems. Physical access to government health facilities in India was also poor. In Sri Lanka, problems within the health sector were not perceived to be as acute: geographical and financial access to government facilities and availability of staff inputs were good. However, government officials feared that dwindling resources might threaten the effectiveness of what had traditionally been a relatively high performing health sector, and there were problems with the availability of drugs and equipment, long waiting times, poor staff attitudes and bypassing lower-level facilities.

In Ghana a long catalogue of problems was identified including poor geographical coverage, poor quality, inadequate emphasis upon public health and primary care, over-allocation of resources to expensive tertiary facilities, overstaffing, lack of a consumer orientation amongst staff, and inequitable distributions of government subsidies (which were absorbed mainly by facilities in urban areas). Zimbabwe similarly suffered from an overemphasis upon the hospital level, which resulted in users bypassing lower-level facilities. As elsewhere, poor staff motivation and lack of drugs were also problems.

In contrast the Thai health sector performed relatively well: government maintained a high level of geographical coverage and strong government policies on public health issues. Whilst consumer surveys suggested that there was a lack of staff responsiveness to users similar to that found elsewhere, they also indicated that users, particularly inpatients, appreciated the good standards of clinical care in government facilities (Tangcharoensathien 1996). However, centralised and bureaucratic management was considered to reduce efficiency and responsiveness.

There was therefore a perceived need for reform in all the countries – a need perceived by both internal actors and external agencies. Even if there had not been widespread implementation of a reform agenda, to what extent had progress been made with specific reforms?

4.   Specific policy reforms

The research presented in this book chose four tracer policies to study in depth: 1) decentralisation of hospital management; 2) user fees; 3) contracting out to the private sector; and 4) regulation and enabling of the private sector. These were chosen both because they would enable an overview of the policy and implementation of NPM-type reforms, and because they have been the subject of much emphasis in the international literature.

4.1   Progress in implementation

As apparent from earlier chapters, the research found that progress in implementing these policies in practice was very limited in the countries. Table 9.2 summarises the extent of policy implementation in the case-study countries, and visually indicates, through shading, its degree. While Ghana and Zimbabwe had components of a policy reform agenda that bore many hallmarks of NPM, the extent to which this had been implemented was very limited. This was especially true with respect to the principal reforms, for example, implementing a purchaser provider split, contracting out and more generally enabling the private sector. In contrast, much greater progress had been made with implementing a user-fee policy.

However, in some cases these policies existed, but were of relatively long standing and pre-dated the NPM era. This was particularly the case in

Table 9.2 The extent and pace of policy implementation in the case study countries

Selected policies from the NPM agenda	Ghana	Zimbabwe	India (Tamil Nadu)	Sri Lanka	Thailand
User fees	Increased fees implemented Cost recovery c 10 per cent Exemptions to the poor rare	Increased fees implemented Cost recovery c 4 per cent Exemption system weak	No national policy; Fees in some states; not Tamil Nadu	Not on policy agenda	Fees implemented Hospitals recovered c 50 per cent of recurrent costs Relatively effective exemption system
Autonomous hospitals	Legislation passed for teaching hospitals (1988; 1996) Limited implementation	Proposed only, for central and provincial hospitals	No national policy; not on policy agenda of Tamil Nadu	Not on policy agenda; one existed for historical reasons	No policy, though in some respects hospitals enjoyed substantial autonomy due to fee revenue
Clinical contracts	Long-standing subsidies to church facilities	Long-standing subsidies to church facilities	Contracting out of a diagnostic service	Not on policy agenda	Contracting out for some high tech. clinical services and under social insurance scheme
Non-clinical contracts	Policy development stalled	Programme of non-clinical contracting implemented	Traditional tender system for some non clinical services	Traditional tender system for some non clinical services	Widespread non clinical contracting

Table 9.2 (*continued*)

Selected policies from the NPM agenda	Ghana	Zimbabwe	India (Tamil Nadu)	Sri Lanka	Thailand
Deregulation, enablement	Pre-existing liberal stance. Some very limited donor-funded enabling measures implemented	Pre-existing liberal stance. Some very limited donor-funded enabling measures implemented	Tax breaks; liberalisation under discussion for health insurance	Tax breaks	Extensive private sector encouraged by subsidies Compulsory insurance arrangements channelled funding to private providers Recognition of need for strengthened regulatory framework but little progress
Regulation of the private sector	Some revision and extension of laws	Some revision and extension of laws	New regulations enacted but not yet implemented	New legislation being introduced	

Sources: Bennett et al. 1998, Bennett and Muraleedharan 1998, Russell and Attanayake 1997, Russell et al. 1997 and Smithson et al. 1997.

Note: depth of shading indicates the extent to which the selected policies have been implemented.

Thailand, where user fees had been in place for many decades, and where hospitals, because of their very substantial fee revenue which they were allowed to retain, had in practice substantial autonomy over many areas of management. This was also the case for contracting out in the three Asian countries, where it was not uncommon to contract out non-clinical services, for agreements with church providers in Ghana and Zimbabwe, and for the one autonomous hospital in Sri Lanka.

4.2 Performance of new roles

Performance with respect to autonomous hospitals

Due to lack of policy implementation, autonomous hospital policy was largely untested. Researchers were able to identify hospitals which (primarily for historical reasons) had relatively greater autonomy than other facilities, but the difference in levels of autonomy was often slim and the more autonomous hospitals were better funded and had a different clientèle, making it difficult to evaluate the impact of this policy upon performance. There was some evidence to suggest that financial autonomy led to higher structural and input quality, but it appeared that this was often gained at higher cost rather than better management performance or improved technical efficiency.

In a number of instances, policies on autonomy had been adopted as a means to facilitate initiatives for raising resources. Success, however, had been limited. Cost recovery ratios at the two teaching hospitals in Ghana had remained at about 20 per cent, the hospitals were heavily dependent upon MOH funding and in recent years had experienced a growing deficit. APVVP in Andhra Pradesh had experienced considerable political difficulty in implementing user fees, and despite very low charges had eventually withdrawn fees in the face of continuing opposition. Success in revenue raising at the Sri Jayawardenapura General Hospital in Sri Lanka had been greater: fee revenue had accounted for about 30 per cent of income, but the hospital's special position made this possible and this experience could not be applied to other Sri Lankan hospitals.

Success with autonomy appeared to be greater when it was given to organisations engaged in rather less complex tasks, or better defined tasks, and particularly those where there may have been less conflict between equity and commercial objectives. For example, experience with autonomous agencies for drug supply, AIDS control and blindness control in Tamil Nadu all seemed to be relatively positive. There were no pressures on these organisations to recover operating costs through patient fees, and the organisations benefited from freedom from bureaucratic financial controls which gave them the ability to innovate in service organisation.

Performance of user fee implementation

Performance with respect to revenue generation varied. Whilst Ghana had managed to raise approximately 10 per cent of operating costs through fees, in Zimbabwe the comparable figure had not reached 5 per cent. Ghana (like Kenya) was amongst the highest revenue raisers in Sub-Saharan Africa, but still did not compare with Thailand, which had covered approximately 50 per cent of facility-level operating costs through fees. In Ghana, Zimbabwe and Kenya it appeared that due to harsh economic conditions, fee revenue had been used mainly to maintain basic services rather than improve them. However, the introduction of the drug 'cash and carry' system in Ghana appeared to have improved drug availability significantly. In Zimbabwe all revenues from fees had returned to the Ministry of Finance until 1996, reducing incentives to collect revenues and the potential for quality improvements.

There were substantial concerns about the impact of user fees on equity: in both Ghana and Zimbabwe, there had been drops in attendances after the increase in fees. Adverse equity effects had been exacerbated by limited changes in quality and exemption policy failures. Lack of monitoring and evaluation systems for user fees in Ghana and Zimbabwe had meant that it was difficult for authorities to make a reliable assessment of user fee impact, particularly with respect to exemption policy effectiveness, and thus to improve policy implementation.

Performance with respect to contracting out

There had been relatively few problems with specifying and implementing contracts for non-clinical services, with the main problem being a failure to establish quality standards in the contracts. Only Ghana had experienced substantial difficulties in undertaking contracting, and as a consequence contracting plans had developed very slowly. In terms of the performance of the contracts themselves, it seemed that private contractors in the Asian countries could often offer services at lower cost, but that this might entail compromising quality. This is not surprising given the poor specification of quality standards. Most private contractors also had a comparative advantage in terms of staffing: they were tied neither to government pay scales nor to staffing norms, and tended to have lower labour costs. Public sector managers involved in contracting out services appreciated the fact that they were freed from an activity which, whilst essential, was not a core part of their business.

The clinical contracts found were either (a) with non-profit (commonly church) providers and were largely informal, or (b) were for diagnostic services provided by contractors within public hospitals. Experience suggested that both types could work reasonably well: with the former because they shared a very similar mission; and with the latter because the services were relatively straightforward, referral was controlled by public physicians and the contractor had a strong financial interest in maintaining functioning equipment. It is noteworthy that Ministries of Health were generally very cautious about embarking on contracts for clinical care with for-profit providers, feeling that they shared greater common interest with non-profit providers such as church providers and NGOs.

Performance of enabling and regulatory measures

None of the study countries had needed to implement liberalisation within the health sector as all had had a relatively liberal stance already. Several of the governments studied (most notably Ghana) had made vague policy pronouncements about the need for efforts to 'enable' the private sector. None appeared to have moved forward to implement these. Where measures were in place to encourage or strengthen the private sector, with the exception of one specific type of policy, namely subsidies and tax breaks, they tended to be piecemeal, and donor-driven and financed. India, Thailand, and Sri Lanka all had tax-break programmes (largely run out of the MOF or similar body) to encourage private sector growth and these programmes generally included the health sector. Criteria for receiving support were often vague and hence open to manipulation and inappropriate use. Coordination between the organisation responsible for running the subsidy programme and the MOH was generally poor, with neither branch of government monitoring the tax subsidy programme adequately. As a consequence, subsidies granted may have helped to expand the private sector but did not contribute to health sector goals such as improving quality of care or service coverage.

With regard to regulation of the private sector, performance was generally very poor indeed. In all countries studied, there was a patchwork of outdated regulatory statutes which delegated a substantial amount of regulatory authority to professional councils. By and large these councils had proved very imperfect agents for government: they had sorely neglected their duties and in some instances had perverted them to serve their own interests. Governments had neither monitored professional councils nor taken action to encourage them to regulate more effectively. None of the core countries had maintained complete databases of private providers: most were highly incomplete, making regulation impossible. Inspections of private providers had tended to be infrequent and such inspection units appeared prone to corruption.

In all the countries studied, there was concern about the quality of care provided in the private sector. Heterogeneity within the private sector made the picture quite complex: amongst certain providers (e.g. quacks in India and traditional healers in Ghana) there was concern about absolute lack of knowledge. Amongst private providers practising Western medicine, concerns related more to the provision of unnecessary services. These problems may explain why all countries were seeking to improve regulation, though progress appeared very slow.

5.   Relevance of the NPM agenda and related health sector reforms

The research in this book both supports and questions the health sector reform agenda. It supports it in the sense that the country case studies found many of the problems with government performance that the reform agenda was designed to address. These included highly centralised and inefficient systems of management of health services; health care delivery that was unresponsive to clients; services biased to the provision of hospital care and short of vital supplies; and public resource allocation processes that advantaged the better-off more than the poor.

Indeed, Ministries of Health in developing countries frequently epitomise the bureaucratic model of direct service delivery so widely criticised as monopolistic, overcentralised, hierarchical and unresponsive to users. The international health sector reform agenda can be seen as a logical response. However, it is a response which, in the circumstances of the core case study countries, seemed quite out of touch with the reality of their health systems and the broader socio-political environment. The lack of progress with a broader reform agenda and the substantial difficulties faced in both designing and implementing the four policies examined suggest that the problem was not just one of policy design and implementation difficulties, which might be overcome by a sustained capacity building programme (as indeed was done in Kenya for user-fee implementation, and in Zimbabwe for contracting out). Rather there were much more fundamental difficulties and obstacles:

- some NPM-type reforms were inappropriately designed for developing country contexts, and hence even if successfully implemented, may not bring the anticipated benefits;
- the prevailing political and social ethos was antagonistic to the values of NPM in some countries;
- the political feasibility of the reforms was highly questionable, especially in the Asian countries.

Even for those reforms where barriers could be addressed by sustained capacity building, the question remains whether the return to investment in establishing these new roles of government is greater than the return to investment in strengthening the more traditional role of direct provision. In other words, there is a 'value for money' dimension that needs to be considered in deciding on appropriate reform approaches and strategies. These four dimensions of relevance are taken in turn next.

5.1 Design problems

During the research, a number of design features of NPM reforms in the health sector were identified which appeared inappropriate in developing country contexts. For example:

- the extent to which hospitals could be financially autonomous was severely constrained by low ability to pay for hospital care and limited insurance coverage;
- the nature of the livelihoods of the majority of the population meant that much income was in-kind and written evidence of income levels was unavailable: this not only created severe difficulties in designing and implementing exemption mechanisms, but questioned the wisdom of applying user fees among such cash-poor communities;
- contracting out was problematic where the private sector is poorly developed.

Most of the design features which appeared inappropriate were so because of the characteristics of the economic environment, and particularly low levels of market development, and would therefore fall within the definition of capacity used in this research. It is notable from Table 9.2 that the extent of adoption of the selected policies was far greater in Thailand than in the four lower income countries. The section next suggests that differences in political and social ethos do not explain this. Rather it can be argued that the requirements relating to internal and external capacity for the policies to work successfully were present in Thailand to a far greater extent than in the poorer countries.

Two more fundamental difficulties with implementing NPM-type policies in developing country health sectors stem from the combination of the particular characteristics of health care, and developing country environments. First, NPM places emphasis on consumer choice, particularly as a way to make providers more responsive. This requires that consumers have the information to exercise choice wisely, and are able to avoid exploitation by better informed providers. There is abundant evidence in the health sector that consumers are very vulnerable, and make choices that they might not make if better informed. Such problems can be particularly acute in developing country contexts where there is frequently considerable social and economic distance between health workers and the less educated and generally poorer users. For example, user-fee experience in low income countries indicates that fees do not empower users, but rather strengthen the ability of health workers to generate income, either for themselves or for their facility. There is a particular danger that the combination of user fees and hospital autonomy might excessively empower hospital managers, allowing revenue-raising objectives to dominate equity objectives and encouraging overprovision of care. There is already evidence of this happening in developing countries, in particular China (Liu 1999), and there were similar concerns in Ghana, though on a smaller scale, as identified in Chapter 5.

Secondly, principal–agent problems raise major questions over the value of competitive contracts for clinical services with for-profit providers. The outputs of health services are difficult both to specify and monitor, providing substantial leeway for an unscrupulous contractor to exploit its position. In some developing countries such as India, it would seem that the professional ethos among health workers is particularly weak, and there is fairly widespread evidence of opportunistic behaviour. Trust-based and relational contracting involving long-term relationships with suppliers can be seen as a logical response to the difficulties of and uncertainties in measuring health outputs and monitoring health care contractors (Roberts, Le Grand and Bartlett 1998).

Regulation raises very similar difficulties. A major concern is quality of care in the private sector, and on technical grounds, quality of care is very difficult to judge and monitor. Country resistance to deliberately encouraging a much greater pluralism in service delivery, and channelling public funding to private providers, may have its roots in a realistic assessment of the difficulties in health care of controlling opportunistic behaviour. For rich countries with respect to regulation, it has been said that

> the current state must have even more strengths and abilities than its archaic predecessors if it is going to capitalise on the virtuous efficiencies of the market place without suffering the latter's side effects which in humanitarian terms are unacceptable. (Bjorkman and Altenstetter, 1997).

If rich countries doubt their ability to control the adverse consequences of a health market, there is even more reason for poor countries to be cautious. The case studies suggest that little faith was placed either in the ability of regulatory authorities to influence providers, or in consumers' ability to choose wisely (except in Thailand for compulsory insurance). Given the existing problems of quality in much of the private sector and weaknesses in the performance of regulatory agencies, this assessment was probably correct.

5.2 Political and social ethos

New Public Management emerged in developed countries as a response to both ideological changes and fiscal crises (Jackson and Price 1994). During the 1970s, there was a breakdown in the consensus which gave a strong social and economic role to the state. Ideas of market failure, which had justified a strong state role, were challenged by notions of government failure. Governments were not seen as disinterested, but rather as acting in their own interests. In addition, public services were viewed as responsive to professionals' rather than users' needs, technically inefficient and overextended, reaching into areas where the private sector could perform better. The solution was seen to be a considerably reduced role for government, with liberalisation of markets and exposure of welfare services including health to a greater degree of competition and market discipline.

Since NPM and its associated values emerged from social, political and economic changes that occurred during the 1970s and 1980s in developed countries, and especially English-speaking countries including the US, UK, Australia and New Zealand, the question as to whether they represent an appropriate set of values for a very different set of countries is an important one. There are two aspects to this question: first, people's beliefs about the appropriate role of the state; and second, their beliefs about the importance of social solidarity versus individualism.

In many developing countries, there has historically been an emphasis upon the state as the engine of growth and development. The perceived importance of the state in the eyes of the general public was perhaps greatest in countries with a colonial heritage where the state was seen at Independence as the vehicle to achieve both growth and greater equity. In many countries, despite the failure of the state to deliver, this view is still widely held among the population. Amongst the study countries, the emphasis on a strong public role was especially evident in Sri Lanka, but also true even in Thailand where pro-market policies now prevail elsewhere in the economy, and in India, Ghana and Zimbabwe where public health services were perceived to have many deficiencies.

In Sri Lanka, the public health system had widespread support, across all social groups, and had to a considerable extent managed to maintain standards despite economic difficulties. In India, public health services had less widespread public support, but were sustained by a very powerful bureaucracy whose self-interest was bound up with the perpetuation of state control.

In Ghana and Zimbabwe, the tradition of state domination seemed less deeply rooted amongst the policy elite as well as amongst the people at large, and was exposed to much greater strain by economic crisis. The governments were also more vulnerable to influence from outside, less responsive to their citizens' views, and less able to assert their own values and ethos. This helps to account for the greater adoption of NPM-type policies. In the words of a major study of Africa's management institutions:

> the strong centralised government inherited from the colonial period – a government without accountability to civil society, lacking transparency and unregulated by legislative checks and balances – lacked moral legitimacy and bred institutional instability, privatisation of the state, and patrimonial incentives and management. Clientelism has usurped moral and political legitimacy, and political and personal loyalty are regarded more than merit. (Dia 1996)

However, it does not follow that NPM values were widely shared in these countries. In particular, public attitudes to the private sector were still influenced by the persisting ideology of state socialism, as reflected in consumer views that private practitioners' main motives were pecuniary.

In Thailand, economic policies in general were very pro-free market, and this impinged on the health sector through the support for tax-breaks to encourage private sector development. In addition public hospitals, given their substantial user-fee revenue, could be quite entrepreneurial in their behaviour. However, in all other respects, the public health services were sustained by the long tradition of strong and centralised government in Thailand. Hence policies on substantial decentralisation and marketisation of public provision had not made much headway.

NPM has tended to uphold the virtues of private sector management styles (Jackson 1994) and to pay much greater attention to efficiency than equity (Gilson 1999). As Jackson says, 'previous values based upon public administration and serving the public interest have been confronted by an emphasis on market testing, serving individual customers and business planning' (1994: 120). Issues such as the distribution of benefits from public services have tended to be ignored.

Cross-cultural studies of values commonly identify the individualism/ collectivism axis as a key dimension along which cultures differ from each other. Hofstede (1980) described this axis as distinguishing between those cultures which valued loosely knit social relations in which individuals were expected to care only for themselves and their immediate families, versus tightly knit social relations in which individuals were expected to care for a much wider group (such as extended family/clan). Another way of conceptualising this is the extent to which an individual finds meaning through the collectivity and their social relations (Schwarz 1997). In general, developed Anglophone countries where NPM has taken greatest hold have been found to be the most individualistic societies, whereas developing countries, such as those examined here, tend to fall at the opposite end of the scale (Hofstede 1991).

These differences in social values may be a part of the explanation of why NPM has been resisted in some developing country contexts. Certainly in Sri Lanka, as we saw in Chapter 5, 'public action and state responses had politically and socially constructed health care as a public good, a basic right for all citizens'.

5.3 Political feasibility

While there was a mismatch between the values of NPM and those evident in the case study countries, especially Sri Lanka, it was in the area of political feasibility that the relevance of NPM was most obviously challenged. The governments did not in general have the support of key stakeholders to implement a radical health reform agenda. Reform had to be initiated within an existing centralised bureaucratic model of direct service delivery, on which an alliance of vested interests in the interventionist state and its service provision arrangements had been built. Consequently, any radical reform agenda was blocked both by existing state institutions and by vested interests which were suspicious of or opposed to reform.

There was some variation both between policies and between countries. Politicians opposed fees in all case study countries, but in Ghana and Zimbabwe succumbed to economic imperatives and the strong demands of the MOH and MOF, backed by international financial institutions. With the exception of Ghana, national politicians were resistant also to decentralisation, either opposing legislative change or where a law had been passed, resisting actual transfer of power (as in the case of the *Panchayat raj* system in India). Reforms appeared to offer few concrete benefits but many political risks: they challenged long-standing bureaucratic arrangements and interests, made politicians vulnerable to accusations of 'privatisation' and could lead to strikes, public opposition and electoral losses.

Senior bureaucrats commonly resisted decentralisation. In Sri Lanka they used technical capacity constraints at subnational levels to justify limited decentralisation, arguing there would be management failure and corruption if central financial control were loosened. However, it is also likely that at least some were primarily concerned about maintaining their own control over provinces, and a few may have been influenced by the possibility that their own personal financial interests would be adversely affected if control over resources were decentralised.

Health workers were critical policy actors for reform implementation. In India and Sri Lanka, government health workers opposed user fees (on ideological grounds in Sri Lanka; for fear of loss of informal fee revenue in India), and contracting out and hospital autonomy (for fear of job losses). Regulation of the private sector (in which government health workers themselves practised, legally or otherwise) was opposed in India. The medical profession was particularly influential: one of the main reasons why Ghana moved ahead with fees and decentralisation was that the MOH and medical professionals led the reform process. In contrast in Sri Lanka, the Government Medical Officers Association consistently opposed decentralisation, which was seen to represent 'implementation of a failed system of autonomy from a developed country'.

Overall, there was little enthusiasm for NPM reforms among key national policy actors in the countries in South Asia, although in India interest might have been greater if broader bureaucratic constraints to reform (such as personnel regulations) were lifted. In the African countries caution and opposition were also widespread, but a key catalyst for reform was deeper economic crisis and a near collapse in service delivery which strengthened pressure for change from internal and external actors. In most of the countries, the push for change came largely from an alliance between a few MOH technocrats and external technical advisors; as a result policy discussions used the 'right' language, but masked major difficulties with implementation.

Given this political environment, the research identified few routes – other than the somewhat unhelpful one of severe economic collapse – to achieving radical policy reforms. Contracting out of non-clinical services in Zimbabwe was one example, where attention to workers' interests seem to have permitted policy implementation. This is perhaps a key point, however: successful implementation of reform programmes commonly entails a weakening of public sector unions (so that workers can be fired, wages set locally, etc.), and an erosion of professional autonomy. In most of the study countries, governments appeared very reluctant to try to wrest power from either public sector unions or professionals (particularly doctors), who were very ready to use strike action to press their demands and/or preserve their position. At the same time, the management cadre in the public sector, probably the only group of workers that might have clearly seen personal benefits from reform programmes, was often very weak and thin. This represents a key difference with the context of NPM reforms in the health sector in developed countries, where changes to strengthen the influence of managers could build on an already strong and capable cadre or recruit them from outside, and indeed a key difference from the implementation of NPM in the UK, where the health service reforms followed on from a period when trade union rights were severely curtailed, and were associated with a general trend to challenge the autonomy of professionals in a number of sectors (Ferlie et al. 1996).

Of considerable relevance in further explaining policy stagnation in a situation where the public heath sector was unsatisfactory was the lack of pressure for change from the general population in the core case study countries. Users were uninvolved in services, in some cases alienated from them, and moreover saw reforms as a threat rather than an opportunity. Extensive use was made of private health services by all groups of the population; thus 'exit' rather than 'voice' was the approach followed, though in the last resort there was greater faith in the public sector to treat severe disease and to behave ethically. Thailand illustrated the potential for greater civil society involvement. Although reforms were not yet really addressing the need for consumer voice, an increasingly active media was beginning to speak on behalf of disadvantaged individuals and groups, and to exert pressure for change on the government bureaucracy.

5.4   Value for money

Even if it is feasible to expand capacity – whether external or internal – to implement the new arrangements discussed in this book, to what extent is that a sensible investment strategy? The key comparison is between the efficiency gains to be anticipated from reforms, and the costs of both bringing them about and of operating them.

Although very little evidence is available about the costs of implementing reform in the health sector of developing countries, evidence from industrialised countries suggests that there can be significant costs associated with transition processes. For example the British government in the period 1992–5 spent at least $512 million on management consultants alone, with the aim of implementing public sector reforms

(*The Economist* 1996). Social costs may also be incurred due to confusion and lower quality care during the transition phase.

Another major concern with many of the NPM reforms has been increased transactions costs with the new service arrangements. The UK health service reforms attracted much publicity for the increased numbers and salaries of managers as well as the costs of new information systems, particularly those required for pricing services, when it moved to a system of contracts for organising service delivery. In contrast, the benefits of the reforms, whether in terms of improved efficiency, responsiveness to users, or cost contain-ment, have been hard to substantiate (Bartlett, Roberts and Le Grand 1998).

Evidence on transaction costs is as yet extremely patchy from developing countries, whether from the case studies in this book or from the literature more generally. The evidence on contracting out of non-clinical services suggests that efficiency gains may in certain circum-stances outweigh any additional transactions costs, but evidence is very limited (Mills 1998). Indeed, a major problem is that insufficient resources are often devoted to managing the new arrangements, whether in relation to strengthening the resources of the purchaser in the case of contracting, or of the regulator in relation to encouraging greater private sector involvement. The result is not only low transactions costs but also poor performance of the new arrangements.

6.   Conclusions

The above discussion implies that radical and wide-ranging reform on NPM lines is not an appropriate strategy for countries such as the low income countries studied here. Certainly evidence from the core case study countries and elsewhere suggests the scope for things to go wrong. For example, where user fees provide revenue to hospitals but without monitoring and control systems in place, broader community oversight, or adequate staff salaries, the hospital is made a key stakeholder in generating income, and concerns of the impact on the poor are ignored. Chinese experience demonstrates the damage this can do to access to health care (World Bank 1997). And where contracting out is introduced without the capacity to manage and monitor contracts, the result can be high-cost, low-quality care as the experience of contracting for primary care in South Africa demonstrates (Kinghorn 1996).

The conclusion of the previous chapter was that where performance is poor and capacity weak, the desirable response is a process of gradual and carefully phased reform. A carefully planned capacity building pro-gramme would encompass skills to manage the transition process and ensure that reforms have widespread support, strengthening of basic administrative systems, gradual change of the organisational culture, and targeted strategies to relieve crucial external capacity constraints. However, the appropriate balance is still unresolved between gradual incremental change on a few fronts which only gradually challenges existing arrangements, and more major reform that may in the shorter run create some degree of chaos but in the longer run can shake up the system and change traditional styles of working.

Whichever approach is attempted, reform needs to be seen as a long term process. It seems often to be forgotten that the UK health service reforms, for example, built on decades of management strengthening and creation of information systems. Thus the capacities existed to take on the required roles, and develop and adapt them to the local context. Where such local capacities are weak and poorly developed, reforms must inevitably be less ambitious.

If the full NPM agenda is not appropriate to low-income countries, what is the alternative? Interestingly, the recent health policy statement of the Asian Development Bank calls for governments to play an appropriate and activist role in the health sector, involving increased central government funding for health, avoidance where possible of user fees for primary care, greater collaboration with the private sector though not as a means for governments to decrease their investments or interest in the health sector, stronger regulation of the private sector, careful experimentation with new forms of service delivery such as contracting out through pilot experiments, and efforts to increase government managerial capacity in both service delivery and policy development and implementation (ADB 1999). There is no emphasis either on competitive strategies or enabling measures. Given the major shocks provided to a number of Asian countries by the financial crisis, and its impact on reducing the demand for private services and expanding the demand for public services, this policy statement possibly reflects the beginnings of a more realistic assessment of what the private sector can do and what governments must do, and how they can best go about it.

However, the international literature is in general remarkably thin in offering alternative models for health sector reform, with the battle-lines drawn between those espousing NPM reforms and those supporting a traditional public sector, monopolistic approach. Ideas are notably absent on how to reform what already exists rather than developing new forms of service delivery. While the research reported here does not provide a comprehensive alternative agenda for health sector reform, it does provide pointers towards such an alternative agenda.

With respect to the process of reform design, appropriate reforms very clearly do need to be context-specific and rooted in a detailed assessment not only of existing organisational structures but also of the broader institutional context. Reforms also need to be more cognisant of the external environment, both constraints embedded in the public sector (such as MOF financial regulations) and broader socio-economic factors. Very frequently NPM-style reforms envisage a quite different set of social relations to those which exist in many low income countries (Flynn 1999). While reforms may want to move away from systems run on the basis of patronage and family connections, it needs to be recognised that this cannot be a short-term agenda.

It is tempting to think that many of the implementation problems apparent in the study countries could have been avoided if there had been greater broad-based ownership of reforms, going beyond a small number of technocrats and donor agencies. Health workers are an obvious group who need to be better informed and more involved during the design phases of reform programmes. In addition, appropriate design of reforms is surely rooted in a clear understanding of what beneficiaries want from reform. The general public must be much better informed on reforms and more deeply involved both in their design and also in the ongoing operation of health services. This requires much greater attention to appropriate ways of involving the general public, including structures and institutions which give poor people access and influence.

Given the existing structure of health systems in most developing countries, reforms which focus upon improving the effectiveness and efficiency of the purely public sector (such as promoting autonomy and management strengthening) and of the purely private sector (such as improved regulation and enabling) would seem to be of higher priority than encouraging government to take on new and complex functions (such as contracting for clinical care). In some countries with very weak capacity, an emphasis upon basic systems (such as establishment of adequate management information systems, enhancing skills of managers, creating greater financial accountability) should be given top priority. Such systems are necessary regardless of the form of service organisation adopted. However the research also found that, in some instances, reforms were hindered by an organisational culture which emphasised adherence to rules and regulations rather than a performance orientation. Organisational culture needs as much attention in a reform programme as organisational structure.

Finally, there appears to be some evidence that the values inherent in NPM conflict with the values held by both the general public and health workers in many developing countries. The cultures of developing countries are more likely to emphasise the collectivity, social solidarity and the welfare of all rather than the individual (Hofstede 1991, Schwarz 1997). Several of the NPM reforms (such as user fees and potentially autonomous hospitals) would seem to exacerbate inequities. Reforms which build upon social solidarity, rather than undermine it, may receive wider support within countries.

Notes

Chapter 1

1. For a brief overview of the forms of market failure most typically associated with health markets, see the annex to this chapter.
2. Existence and timing of structural adjustment was a key consideration since it often initiated a process of government-wide reform in countries (though the extent to which different sectors were affected could vary widely).
3. Separate volumes covering the findings of each of these sector studies are forthcoming.
4. A companion volume (Batley et al. in preparation) will integrate the findings from the four sector studies.

Chapter 2

1. Reimbursement rules and levels were recently restricted following the financial crisis in order to contain costs.
2. To aid interpretation, the graphs have been standardised so that above the line represents better performance and below the line, worse performance.

Chapter 3

1. Though in India in the nineteenth century, the colonial government was careful to distance itself from evangelism, and missionary medicine was much less important than state medicine (Arnold 1988).
2. Interestingly, the Colonial Office had requested it be banned in 1946, and from then on it was severely restricted (Addae 1996).

Chapter 4

1. This privilege was subsequently extended to all hospitals.
2. Peradeniya Teaching Hospital (PTH).
3. Patients lying on mattresses on the floor because of overcrowding.

Chapter 5

1. The two teaching hospitals got around this problem by securing increases in non-drug fee levels in 1990.
2. In Ghana, donors had only recently become involved in strengthening financial management capacity.
3. The SDF, established in 1992 and administered by the DOSW, was one component of the Social Dimensions of Adjustment programme implemented to protect the poor from the harsh economic impact of structural adjustment.

Chapter 6

1. Public providers were to be treated in a similar way, with performance contract agreements with district and regional hospitals and the Ghana Health Service.
2. A flat rate payment per insured person per year, covering virtually all care needed.
3. Though in order to gain experience, the first contracting arrangements were set up in a new hospital where no conflict with existing workers would occur.
4. It is also likely that other reforms, notably restructuring and decentralisation, were higher up their agenda.

Chapter 7

1. The Zimbabwe health sector case study conducted for this research did not address regulation or enabling issues, as simultaneous to this study a more in-depth study of health sector regulation in Zimbabwe was being implemented with overlapping research staff. Most of the references to Zimbabwe in this chapter draw upon this parallel study conducted by Hongoro et al. (1998).
2. Regulations in certain states in India (e.g. Maharastra) did not permit this for doctors of all ranks. However, these regulations were widely flouted and private practice by government doctors was usual throughout India.

Chapter 8

1. It might also be argued that donor dominance is a cause of weak strategic direction in government: if scarce government resources are pulled in different directions by donors, this may impede the development of a broader strategic vision.
2. See Tendler (1997) for some examples where government practice and policy did contribute to very specific organisational cultures.
3. In India the AIDS Control and Blindness Control Societies, and Tamil Nadu Medical Supplies Corporation, fell into this category, and the plans in Ghana to establish a Ghanaian Health Service had a similar character.
4. See in particular Hildebrand and Grindle (1994) for very detailed suggestions on how to promote capacity building, both in terms of the external environment and internal capacity.

Chapter 9

1. Although much of the health status gain is probably attributable to factors outside of the health sector, such as women's literacy, water and sanitation, and food subsidies.
2. With the notable exception of Kerala and increasingly other Southern states such as Tamil Nadu.

References

ADB (Asian Development Bank) (1999) *Policy for the Health Sector*. Asian Development Bank, Manila.

Addae, S. (1997) *The Evolution of Modern Medicine in a Developing Country: Ghana 1880–1960*. Durham Academic Press, Durham.

Advani, R. (1991) *Patients Know Your Rights*. Consumer Education and Research Centre, Ahmedabad.

Aitken, J. (1994) Voices from the inside: managing district health services in Nepal. *International Journal of Health Planning and Management* 9: 309–40.

Alailima, P. and Mohideen, F. (1984) Health sector expenditure flows in Sri Lanka. *World Health Statistics Quarterly* 37(4): 403–20.

Allsopp, J. and Mulcahy, L. (1996) *Regulating Medical Work: Formal and Informal Controls*. Open University Press, Buckingham.

AM90s (African Management in the 1990s) (1994) *From Transplant Approaches to Institutional Reconciliation*. Report drafted for Africa's Management in the 90s Workshop, Dakar, Senegal, 26–29 September. Capacity Building and Implementation Division, Africa Technical Department, World Bank, Washington, DC.

Anderson, B. (1983) *Imagined Communities*. Verso, London.

Arnold, D. (1988) Introduction: disease, medicine and empire. In Arnold, D. (ed.) *Imperial Medicine and Indigenous Societies*. Manchester University Press, Manchester.

Ayee, J.R.A. (1997) The adjustment of central bodies to decentralisation: the case of the Ghanaian bureaucracy. *African Studies Review*, 40: 37–57.

Barnum, H. and Kutzin, J. (1993) *Public Hospitals in Developing Countries: Resource Use, Cost, Financing*. Johns Hopkins University Press, Baltimore.

Barnum, H, Kutzin, J. and Saxenian, H. (1995) Incentives and provider payment methods. *International Journal of Health Planning and Management* 10: 23–45.

Bartlett, W., Roberts, J. and Le Grand, J. (1998) The development of quasi-markets in the 1990s. In Bartlett, W., Roberts, J. and Le Grand, J. (eds) *A Revolution in Social Policy*. The Policy Press, Bristol.

Batley, R. (1997) A *Research Framework for Analysing Capacity to Undertake the 'new' roles of Government*. The Role of Government in Adjusting Economies Paper number 23, University of Birmingham, Birmingham.

Bennett, S. (1997a) The nature of competition among private hospitals in Bangkok, in Bennett, S., McPake, B. and Mills, A. (eds). *Private Health Providers in Developing Countries: Serving the Public Interest?* Zed Press, London.

Bennett, S. (1997b) Private health care and public policy objectives. In Colclough, C. (ed.) *Marketizing Education and Health in Developing Countries. Miracle or Mirage?* Oxford, Clarendon Press.

Bennett, S. (1991) *The Mystique of Markets: Public and Private Health Care in Developing Countries*. Department of Public Health and Policy publication number 4, London School of Hygiene and Tropical Medicine, London.

Bennett, S. and Franco, L. (1999) *Public Sector Health Worker Motivation and Health Sector Reform: A Conceptual Framework*. Partnerships for Health Reform, Abt Associates, Bethesda.

Bennett, S. and Mills, A. (1998) Government capacity to contract: health sector experience and lessons. *Public Administration and Development*, 18: 307–26.

Bennett, S. and Muraleedharan, V.R. (1998) *Reforming the Role of Government in the Tamil Nadu Health Sector*. The Role of Government in Adjusting Economies Paper No. 28, Development Administration Group, University of Birmingham.

Bennett, S. and Ngalande-Banda, E. (1994) *Public and Private Roles in Health: A Review and Analysis of Experience in Sub-Saharan Africa*. SHS Paper No. 6, Division of Strengthening of Health Services, World Health Organisation.

Bennett, S., McPake, B. and Mills, A. (1997) The public/private debate in health care. In Bennett, S., McPake, B. and Mills, A. (eds) *Private Health Providers in Developing Countries: Serving the Public Interest?* Zed Press, London.

Bennett, S., Russell, S. and Mills, A. (1996) *Institutional and Economic Perspectives on Government Capacity to Assume New Roles in the Health Sector: A Review of Experience*. Department of Public Health and Policy publication No. 22, London School of Hygiene and Tropical Medicine, London.

Bennett, S., Mills, A., Russell, S., Supachutikul, A. and Tangcharoensathien, V. (1998) *The Health Sector in Thailand*. Role of government in adjusting economies publication No. 31, Development Administration Group, University of Birmingham.

Beracochea, E. (1997) Contracting out of non-clinical services: the experience of Papua New Guinea. In Bennett, S., McPake, B. and Mills, A. (eds) *Private Health Providers in Developing Countries: Serving the Public Interest?*. Zed Press, London.

Berman, P. (1995) Health sector reform: making health development sustainable. In Berman P. (ed.) *Health Sector Reform in Developing Countries: Making Development Sustainable*. Harvard School of Public Health, Boston.

Bhat, R. (1999) Characteristics of private medical practice in India: a provider perspective. *Health Policy and Planning* 14(1): 26–37.

Bhatia, M. and Mills, A. (1997) The contracting out of dietary services by public hospitals in Bombay. In Bennett, S., McPake, B., and Mills, A. (eds) *Private Health Providers in Developing Countries: Serving the Public Interest?*. Zed Press, London.

Bikales, W.G. (1997) Capacity building in a transition country: lessons from Mongolia. In Grindle, M. (ed.) *Getting Good Government: Capacity Building in the Public Sectors of Developing Countries*. Harvard University Press, Cambridge, MA.

Birdsall, N. and James, E. (1992) *Health, Government and the Poor: The Case for the Private Sector*. World Bank, Policy Research Working Paper No. 938, Washington DC.

Björkman, J.W. and Altenstetter, C. (1997) Globalised concepts and local practice: convergence and divergence in national health policy reforms. In Altenstetter, C., and Björkman, J.W. (eds.) *Health Policy Reform, National Variations and Globalisation*. Macmillan, Basingstoke.

Booth, D., Milimo, J. and Bond, G. et al. (1995) *Coping with Cost Recovery: A Study of the Social Impact of and Response to Cost Recovery in Basic Services (Health and Education) in Poor Communities in Zambia*. Report to SIDA, Commissioned through the Development Studies Unit, Department of Social Anthropology, Stockholm University.

Brinkerhoff, D.W. (1994) Institutional development in World Bank projects: analytical approaches and intervention designs. *Public Administration and Development* 14: 135–51.

Broomberg, J. (1994) Managing the health care market in developing countries: prospects and problems. *Health Policy and Planning* 9, 237–51.

Cammack, P. (1988) *Third World Politics*. Macmillan, Basingstoke.

Cassells, A. (1995) Health sector reform: key issues in less developed countries. *Journal of International Development* 7(3): 329–48.

Cassells, A. and Janovsky, K. (1996). *Reform of the Health Sector in Ghana and Zambia*. Current Concerns SHS paper No. 11, WHO, Geneva.

Chawla, M. and George, A. (1996) *Hospital Autonomy in India: The Experience of APVVP Hospitals*. Data for Decision-Making Project, Harvard School of Public Health, Boston.

CHP and HEU (1999) *Analysing the Process of Health Financing Reform: South Africa Country Report*, (Draft) Centre for Health Policy, University of Witwatersrand and Health Economics Unit, University of Cape Town.

Collins, D., Quick, J., Musau, S. et al. (1996) *Health Financing Reform in Kenya: The Fall and Rise of Cost Sharing, 1989–94*. Management Sciences for Health, Boston.

Cripps, G. (1997) *Resource Allocation Data*. Ministry of Health and Family Welfare, Harare.

Daura, M. et al. (1999) *The SAZA Study: Analysing the Process of Health Financing Reform. Country Report* (draft). Zambia. University of Zambia.

Dia, M. (1996) *Africa's Management in the 1990s and Beyond. Reconciling Indigenous and Transplanted Institutions*. The World Bank, Washington, DC.

Donaldson, C. and Gerard, K. (1993) *Economics of Health Care Financing: The Visible Hand*. Macmillan, Basingstoke.

Drèze, J. and Sen, A. (1989) *Hunger and Public Action*. Clarendon Press, Oxford.

Duggal, R. (1997) Health care budgets in a changing political economy. *Economic and Political Weekly* 32(20–21): 1197–200.

Dummett, R. (1993) Disease and mortality amongst gold miners of Ghana: colonial government and mining company attitudes and policies 1900–1938. *Social Science and Medicine* 37(2): 213–32.

Ellis, R.P., Alam, M. and Gupta, I. (1996) Health insurance in India: prognosis and prospectus. Boston University, unpublished.

Ensor, T. and San, P. (1996) Access and payment for health care: the poor of Vietnam. *International Journal of Health Planning and Management*, 11: 69–83.

Ernst and Young (1994) Current Financing of Health Care in Sri Lanka and its Implications. Mimeo. Colombo, Sri Lanka.

Ferlie, E., Ashburner, A., Fitzerald, A., and Pettigrew, A. (1996) *The New Public Management in Action*. Oxford University Press, Oxford.

Fiszbein, A. (1997) The emergence of local capacity: lessons from Colombia. *World Development* 25(7): 1029–43.

Flynn, N. (1999) *Comments*. Role of Government Conference, Birmingham, March 1999.

Forster, C. (1994) *Contracting out Ancillary Services: Applying the UK Experience*. Ministry of Health/ODA, Accra, Ghana.

Gilson, L. (1999) Re-addressing equity: the importance of ethical processes. In Mills, A. (ed.) *Reforming Health Sectors*. Kegan Paul, London.

Gilson, L. (1997) The lessons of user fee experience in Africa. *Health Policy and Planning*, 12(4): 273–85.

Gilson, L. and Mills, A. (1995) Health sector reforms in Sub-Saharan Africa: lessons of the last 10 years. In Berman, P. (ed.) *Health Sector Reform in Developing Countries: Making Health Development Sustainable*. Harvard School of Public Health, Boston.

Gilson, L., Russell, S. and Buse, K. (1995) The political economy of user fees with targeting: developing equitable health financing policy. *Journal of International Development*, 7(3): 369–401.

Gilson, L., Adusei, J., Arhin, D. et al. (1997) Should governments in developing countries contract out clinical services to NGOs? In Bennett, S., McPake, B. and Mills, A. (eds) *Private Health Providers in Developing Countries: Serving the Public Interest?*. Zed Press, London.

Gilson, L., Russell, S., Rauyajin, O. et al. (1998) *Exempting the Poor: A Review and Evaluation of the Low Income Card Scheme in Thailand*. Department of Public Health and Policy Publication No. 30, London School of Hygiene and Tropical Medicine, London.

Government of India (1997) *Fifth Conference of the Central Council of Health and Family Welfare*. Ministry of Health and Family Welfare, New Delhi.

Government of the Republic of Zimbabwe (1981) *Planning for Equity in Health*. Government Printing Office, Harare.

Grant, K. and Beach, I. (1994) Report of a strategic review of the Health Management Strengthening Project provided for the Government of Zimbabwe by the Overseas Development Administration of the United Kingdom, December.

Green, A. (1997) *Health Sector Reform: Policy Formulation and Implementation*. Country Report on Thailand. Nuffield Institute for Health, Leeds.

Griffin, C. (1992) Welfare gains from user charges for government health services. *Health Policy and Planning*, 7(2): 177–80.

Griffin, C., Levine, R. and Eakin, K. (1994) *Government and Private Health Care Facilities in Sri Lanka*. The Urban Institute, Washington, DC.

Grindle, M. (1997) Divergent cultures? When public organisations perform well in developing countries. *World Development* 25(4): 481–95.

Grindle, M. and Hildebrand, M. (1995) Building sustainable capacity in the public sector: what can be done? *Public Administration and Development*, 15: 441–63.

GSS (Ghana Statistical Service) (1995) *Ghana Living Standards Survey – Report on the Third Round (GLSS3): September 1991 – September 1992*. Ghana Statistical Service, Accra.

Haque, M.S. (1998) Legitimation crisis: a challenge for public service in the next century. *International Review of Administrative Sciences* 64: 13–26.

Harding, A. and Preker, A. (1999) Conceptual framework. In *Innovations in Health Care Delivery: Organisational Reforms within the Public Sector* (draft). The World Bank, Washington DC.

Hecht, R., Overholt, C. and Holmberg, H. (1993) Improving the implementation of cost recovery: lessons from Zimbabwe. *Health Policy*, 25: 213–42.

Herbst, J. (1993) *The Politics of Reform in Ghana, 1982–91*. University of California Press, Berkeley.

Hildebrand, M.E. and Grindle, M.S. (1994) *Building Sustainable Capacity: Challenges for the Public Sector*. UNDP and HIID, Harvard University, Cambridge.

Hirschmann, D. (1993) Institutional development in the era of economic policy reform: concerns, contradictions and illustrations from Malawi. *Public Administration and Development* 13: 113–28.

Hofstede, G. (1991) *Cultures and Organizations: Software of the Mind*. McGraw-Hill, New York.

Hofstede, G. (1980) *Culture's Consequences: International Differences in Work-related Values*. Sage, Beverly Hills, CA.

Hongoro, C. and Chandiwana, S. (1994) *The Effects of User Fees on Health Care Delivery in Zimbabwe*. Blair Research Institute, MOHCW and UNICEF.

Hongoro, C., Kumanarayake, Chirove J. and Musonza, T. (1998) Regulation of the private health sector in Zimbabwe. Draft, Health Economics and Financing Programme, London School of Hygiene and Tropical Medicine, London.

IDS Health Group (1978) *Health Needs and Health Services in rural Ghana*, Vol. 1. Institute of Development Studies, Brighton.

India Today (1995) Doctors: Holding them to account. *India Today* 15 December.

Inter-American Development Bank (1996) *Economic and Social Progress in Latin America*. Special section 'Making Social Services Work'. Washington, DC: Johns Hopkins University Press for the Inter-American Development Bank.

Jackson, P.M. (1994) The new public sector management: surrogate competition and contracting out. In Jackson, P.M. and Price, C. (eds) *Privatisation and Regulation: A Review of the Issues*. Longman, London.

Jackson, P.M. and Price, C.M. (1994) Privatisation and regulation: A review of the issues. In Jackson, P.M. and Price, C.M. *Privatisation and Regulation: A Review of the Issues*, Longman, New York.

Jalan, J. and Subbaarao, K. (1995) Adjustment and social sectors in India. In Cassen, R. and Joshi, V. (ed.) *India: The Future of Economic Reform*. Oxford University Press, Delhi.

Jarrett, S. and Ofosu-Amaah, S. (1992) Strengthening health services for MCH in Africa: the first four years of the Bamako Initiative. *Health Policy and Planning*, 7(2): 164–76.

Jesani, A. (1996) *Laws and Health Care Providers: A Study of Legislation and Legal Aspects of Health Care Delivery*. CEHAT, Bombay.

Kalumba K (1997) *Towards an Equity-oriented Policy of Decentralisation in Health Systems under Conditions of Turbulence: The Case of Zambia*. Forum on Health Sector Reform, Discussion Paper No. 6, World Health Organisation, Geneva.

Kanji, N. and Jazdowska, N. (1993) Structural adjustment and women in Zimbabwe. *Review of African Political Economy*. 56: 11–26.

Kaul, M. (1997) The New Public Administration: management innovations in government. *Public Administration and Development* 17: 13–26.

Kinghorn, A. (1996) *The Role of General Practitioners in a Future National Health System: Experience with Contracting of Part-time District Surgeons and Suggestions for Change*. Centre for Health Policy, Johannesburg.

Klages, H. and Loffler, E. (1998) New Public Management in Germany: the implementation process of the New Steering Model. *International Review of Administrative Sciences* 64: 41–54.

Klitgaard, R. (1988) *Controlling Corruption*. University of California Press, Berkeley.

Knowles, J. (1997) *Indicators of Health Sector Reform*. Partnerships for Health Reform Project, Abt Associates, Bethesda.

Korboe, D. (1995) *Extended Poverty Study: Access and Utilisation of Basic Social Services by the Poor in Ghana*. Report commissioned by UNICEF.

Kutzin, J. (1995) *Experience with Organisational and Financing Reform of the Health Sector*. Current Concerns SHS Paper No. 8, WHO/SHS/CC94.3. World Health Organisation, Geneva.

Lalta, S. (1993) *Cost Containment and Competitive Tendering for Support Services in the Health Care System of Jamaica*. Institute of Social and Economic Research, University of the West Indies, Jamaica.

Larbi, G. (1998) Institutional constraints and capacity issues in decentralising management in public services: the case of health in Ghana. *Journal of International Development*, 10: 377–86.

Leighton, C. (1996) Strategies for achieving health financing reform in Africa. *World Development* 24(9): 1511–25.

Lennock, J. (1994) *Paying for Health: Poverty and Structural Adjustment in Zimbabwe*. Oxfam Insight. Oxfam Publications, Oxford.

Liu, X. (1999)) *Impact of Payment Reforms to Hospital-based Doctors in the Efficiency of Hospital Services. A Study of Country General Hospitals in China.* PhD thesis, University of London.

Londono, J. and Frenk, J. (1997) Structured pluralism: Towards a new model of health system reform in Latin America. *Health Policy* 41: 1–36.

Mackintosh, M. (1997) *Informal Regulation: A Conceptual Framework and Application to Decentralised Mixed Finance in Health Care.* Paper prepared for the conference on Public Sector Management for the Next Century, Institute of Development Policy and Management, Manchester, 29 June–2 July.

Mackintosh, M. (1995) Competition and contracting in selective social provisioning. *European Journal of Development Research* 7: 26–52.

Mackintosh, M. (1992) Questioning the state. In Wuyts, M., Mackintosh, M. and Hewitt, T. (eds) *Development Policy and Public Action*. Oxford University Press, Oxford.

Marmor, T.R. (1997) Global health policy reform. In Altenstetter, C., and Björkman, J.W. (eds) *Health Policy Reform, National Variations and Globalisation*. Macmillan, Basingstoke.

Maynard, A. (1982) The regulation of public and private health care markets. In McLachlan, G. and Maynard, A. (eds) *The Public/Private Mix Debate for Health: The Relevance and Effects of Change*. Nuffield Provincial Hospitals Trust, London.

McNaught, A. and Lazarus, J. (1994) *Report on Hospital Management Consultancy*. Ministry of Health, Ghana.

McPake, B. (1996) Public autonomous hospitals in sub-Saharan Africa. *Health Policy* 35: 155–77.

McPake, B. and Hongoro, C. (1995) Contracting out of clinical services in Zimbabwe. *Social Science and Medicine* 41(1), 13–24.

McPake, B. and Hongoro, C. (1993) *Contracting-out in Zimbabwe: A Case Study of a Contract between Wankie Colliery Hospital and the Ministry of Health*. Health Economics and Financing Programme, London School of Hygiene and Tropical Medicine.

McPake, B and Kutzin, J. (1997) *Methods for Evaluating Effects of Health Reforms*. Division of Analysis, Research and Assessment, WHO, Geneva.

Mills, A. (1998) To contract or not to contract? Issues for low and middle income countries. *Health Policy and Planning* 13(1): 32–40.

Mills, A (1997a) Improving the efficiency of public sector health services in developing countries: bureaucratic versus market approaches. In Colclough, C. (ed.) *Marketising Education and Health in Developing Countries*. Clarendon Press, Oxford.

Mills, A. (1997b) Contractual relationships between government and the commercial private sector in developing countries. In Bennett, S., McPake, B. and Mills, A. (eds). *Private Health Providers in Developing Countries: Serving the Public Interest?* Zed Press, London.

Mills, A. and Broomberg, J. (1998) *Experiences of Contracting: An Overview of the Literature.* Macroeconomics, Health and Development Series, No. 33. World Health Organisation, Geneva.

Mills, A., Bennett, S., Siriwanarangsun, Tangcharoensathien, V. (2000) The response of providers to capitation payment: a case-study from Thailand. *Health Policy.* 51: 163-180

Mills, A., Vaughan, J.P., Smith, D.L. and Tabibzadeh, I. (1990) *Health System Decentralisation: Concepts, Issues and Country Experience.* World Health Organisation, Geneva.

Ministry of Health, Sri Lanka (1996) *National Health Policy,* Ministry of Health, Colombo.

MOHCW, Zimbabwe (1996) *Proposals for Health Sector Reform.* Ministry of Health and Child Welfare, Harare.

Ministry of Public Health, Thailand (1997) *Health in Thailand 1995–6.* Bureau of Health Policy and Plan, Ministry of Public Health, Thailand.

Ministry of Public Health, Thailand (1992) *The Seventh Five Year National Health Development Plan (1992–1996).* Health Planning Division, Ministry of Public Health, Bangkok.

Ministry of Health, Ghana (1995) *Medium Term Health Strategy: Towards Vision 2020.* Ministry of Health, Accra.

Ministry of Health, Ghana (1998) Contracting with private health sector providers. Memorandum of Understanding. Ministry of Health, Accra.

Møgedal, S., Steen, S.H. and Mpelumbe, G. (1995) Health sector reform and organisational issues at the local level: lessons from selected African countries. *Journal of International Development,* 7(3): 349–67.

MOHCW, Zimbabwe (1996) *Proposals for Health Sector Reform.* Ministry of Health and Child Welfare, Harare, Zimbabwe.

Moran, M. and Wood, B. (1993) *States, Regulation and the Medical Profession.* Open University Press, Buckingham.

Morgan, P. (1999) *An Update on the Performance Monitoring of Capacity Development Programs: What Are We Learning?* Paper presented at the meeting of the DAC Informal Network on Institutional and Capacity Development, Ottawa, 3–5 May.

Morgan, G. (1986) Creating social reality: organisations as cultures. In *Images of Organisation.* Sage Publications, Newbury Park.

Mudyarabikwa, O. (1999) *Assessment of Incentive Setting for Participation of Private For-profit Health Care Providers in Zimbabwe.* Partnerships for Health Reform, Abt Associates, Bethesda.

Muraleedharan, V.R. (1999) *Characteristics and Structure of the Private Hospital Sector in Urban India: a study of Madras City.* Small Applied Research Paper No. 5, Partnerships for Health Reform Project, Abt Associates, Bethesda.

Musgrove, P. (1996) *Public and Private Roles in Health: Theory and Financing Patterns.* World Bank Discussion Paper No. 339, World Bank, Washington DC.

Mutizwa-Mangiza, D. (1998) *Health Sector Reform and Health Worker Motivation in Zimbabwe.* Applied Research Working Paper, Partnerships for Health Reform Project, Abt Associates, Bethesda.

Mutizwa-Mangiza, D. (1997) *The Opinions of Health and Water Service Users in Zimbabwe.* Role of Government in Adjusting Economies Paper number 24, University of Birmingham, Birmingham.

Nittayaramphong, S. and Tangcharoensathien V. (1994) Thailand: private health care out of control? *Health Policy and Planning* 9(1): 31–40.

Nolan, B. and Turbat, V. (1995) *Cost Recovery in Public Health Services in Sub-Saharan Africa*. Economic Development Institute Technical Material. World Bank, Washington DC.

North, D.C. (1990) *Institutions, Institutional Change and Economic Performance*. Cambridge University Press, Cambridge.

Norton, A., Arytee, E.B.-D., Korboe, D. and Dogbe, D.K.T. (1995) *Poverty Assessment in Ghana Using Qualitative and Participatory Research Methods*. Poverty and Social Policy Department Discussion Paper No. 83, World Bank, Washington DC.

Presidential Task Force (1992) *Report of the Presidential Task Force on Formulation of a National Health Policy for Sri Lanka*. Democratic Socialist Republic of Sri Lanka, Government Publications Bureau, Colombo.

OECD (1992) *The Reform of Health Care: A Comparative Analysis of Seven OECD Countries*. Health Policy Studies No. 2. OECD, Paris.

Ofosu Amaah, S. (1981) The maternal and health services in Ghana (their origins and future). *Journal of Tropical Medicine and Hygiene* 84: 256–9.

Osborne, D. and Gaebler, T. (1992) *Reinventing Government: How the Entrepreneurial Spirit is Transforming the Public Sector*. Plume Books, New York.

Ostrom, E., Schroeder, L., and Wynne, S. (1993) *Institutional Incentives and Sustainable Development: Infrastructure Policies in Perspective*. Westview Press, Boulder.

Packard, R.M. (1990) *White Plague, Black Labour, Tuberculosis and the Political Economy of Health and Disease in South Africa*. James Currey, London.

Pandya, S.K. (1994) Letter from Bombay: Why is our food and drugs administration in such poor shape? *The National Medical Journal of India* 7(2): 87–8.

Patterson, K.D. (1981) *Health in Colonial Ghana: Disease, Medicine and Socio-economic Change*. Crossroads Press, Waltham, Mass.

Paul, S. (1995) *Capacity Building for Health Sector Reform*. Forum on Health Sector Reform, WHO, Geneva.

Paul, S. (1992) Accountability in public services: exit, voice and control. *World Development* 20(7): 1047–60.

Private Initiatives for Primary Health Care (1995) *Private Sector Health Care Services in Ghana: Results of a National Survey of Private Health Facilities*. JSI, Research and Training Institute, Arlington, Virginia.

Rakodi, C. (1996) *The Opinions of Health and Water Service Users in Ghana*. Role of Government in Adjusting Economies Paper No. 10, University of Birmingham, Birmingham.

Rakodi, C. (1998) *The Opinions of Health and Water Service Users in India*. Role of Government in Adjusting Economies Paper No. 32, University of Birmingham, Birmingham.

Ramasubban, R. (1982) *Public Health and Medical Research in India: Their Origins under the Impact of British Colonial Policy*. SAREC, Stockholm.

Republic of Sri Lanka (1996) *The National Health Policy*. Democratic Socialist Republic of Sri Lanka.

Roberts, J., Le Grand, J. and Bartlett, W. (1998) Lessons from experience of quasi markets in the 1990s. In Bartlett, W., Roberts, J. and Le Grand, J. (eds) *A Revolution in Social Policy*. The Policy Press, Bristol.

Roth, G. (1988) *The Private Provision of Public Services in Developing Countries*. EDI Series in Economic Development, Oxford University Press, Oxford.

Russell, S. (1996) Ability to pay for health care: concepts and evidence. *Health Policy and Planning*, 11(3): 219–37.

Russell, S. and Attanayake, N. (1997) *Reforming the Health Sector in Sri Lanka: Does Government Have the Capacity?* The Role of Government in Adjusting Economies Paper number 14, Development Administration Group, University of Birmingham.

Russell, S. and Gilson, L. (1997) User fee policies to promote health service access for the poor: a wolf in sheep's clothing? *International Journal of Health Services*, 27 (2): 359–79.

Russell, S. and Gilson, L. (1995) *User Fees at Government Health Services: is Equity Being Considered? An International Survey.* Department of Public Health and Policy Publication No. 15. London School of Hygiene and Tropical Medicine.

Russell, S., Kwaramba, P., Hongoro, C. and Chikandi, S. (1997) *Reforming the Health Sector in Zimbabwe: Does Government Have the Capacity?* The Role of Government in Adjusting Economies Research Programme Paper 20, Development Administration Group, University of Birmingham.

Saltman, R. and Figueras, J. (1997) *European Health Care Reform: Analysis of Current Strategies.* WHO Regional Office for Europe, Copenhagen.

Savedoff, W.D. (1998) Social services viewed through new lenses. In Savedoff W.D. (ed). *Organisation Matters: Agency Problems in Health and Education in Latin America.* Inter-American Development Bank, Washington DC.

Schick, A. (1998) Why most developing countries should not try New Zealand's reforms. *The World Bank Research Observer* 13(1): 123–31.

Schwarz, S. H. (1997) Values and culture. In Munro, D., Schumaker, J. F. and Carr, S.C. (eds) *Motivation and Culture.* Routledge, New York.

Sen, A. (1988) Sri Lanka's achievements: how and when. In Srinivasan, T.N. and Bardhan, P.K. (eds) *Rural poverty in South Asia.* Oxford University Press, Delhi.

Sen, A. (1992) The political economy of targeting. Text of a keynote speech at a conference on 'Public expenditure and the poor: incidence and targeting', at the World Bank, Washington, DC, 17–19 June.

Shaw, P. and Griffin, C. (1995) *Financing Health Care in Sub-Saharan Africa through User Fees and Insurance.* World Bank, Washington DC.

Silva, T., Russell, S. and Rakodi, C. (1997) *The Opinions of Health and Water Service Users in Sri Lanka.* The Role of Government in Adjusting Economies Paper No. 25, Development Administration Group, University of Birmingham.

Smithson, P. (1993) *Sustainability in the Health Sector Part 2: Financial Constraints to Health Service Operation and Development in Ghana.* Save the Children Fund (UK), London.

Smithson, P., Asamoa-Baah, A. and Mills, A. (1997) *The Case of the Health Sector in Ghana.* Role of government in adjusting economies publication No. 26, Development Administration Group, University of Birmingham.

Tangcharoensathien, V. (ed.) (1996) *Payment Mechanisms, Efficiency and Quality of Care in Nine Hospitals in Bangkok.* Report Volume 1. Health Systems Research Institute, Bangkok.

Tangcharoensathien, V. and Supachutikul, A. (1999) The social security scheme in Thailand: what lessons can be drawn? *Social Science and Medicine* 48: 913–24.

Tangcharoensathien, V., Nittayaramphong, S. and Khonsawatt, S. (1997) Contracting out: a case study of public hospitals in Bangkok, Thailand. In Bennett, S., McPake, B. and Mills, A.(eds) *Private Health Providers in Developing Countries: Serving the Public Interest?.* Zed Press, London.

Tangcharoensathien, V., Supachutikul, A. and Nitayarumphong, S. (1992). Cost recovery of hospitals under the Ministry of Public Health. *Chulalongkorn Medical Journal*, 36(8): 593–9.

Tendler, J. (1997) *Good Government in the Tropics.* Johns Hopkins University Press, Baltimore.

The Economist (1996) Leviathian re-engineered. *The Economist,* 19 October, 106.

Tsey, K. and Short, S.D. (1995) From headloading to the iron horse: the unequal health consequences of railway construction and expansion in the Gold Coast 1898–1929. *Social Science and Medicine* 40(5): 613–21.

Twumasi, P.A. (1979) A social history of the Ghanaian pluralistic medical system. *Social Science and Medicine* 13B: 49–56.

UNICEF (1998) *Implementing Health Sector Reforms in Africa: A Review of Eight Country Experiences.* Division of Evaluation, Policy and Planning, UNICEF, New York.

UNICEF (1994) *Children and Women in Zimbabwe: A Situation Analysis.* UNICEF, Harare.

Uplekar, M. (1989a) *Implications of Prescribing Patterns of Private Doctors in the Treatment of Tuberculosis in Bombay, India.* Research Paper No. 41, Takemi Program in International Health, Harvard School of International Public Health, Boston, USA.

Uplekar, M. (1989b) *Private Doctors and Public Health: The Case of Leprosy in Bombay, India.* Research Paper No. 40, Takemi Program in International Health, Harvard School of International Public Health, Boston, USA.

Urageda, C.G. (1987) *A History of Medicine in Sri Lanka from the Earliest Times to 1948.* Sri Lankan Medical Association, Colombo.

Waddington, C.J. and Enyimayew, K.A. (1989) A price to pay: the impact of user charges in Ashanti-Akim District, Ghana. *International Journal of Health Planning and Management* 4: 17–47.

Waddington, C. and Enyimayew, K.A. (1990) A price to pay, part 2: the impact of user charges in the Volta Region of Ghana. *International Journal of Health Planning and Management,* 5: 287–312.

Walsh, K. (1995) *Public Services and Market Mechanisms. Competition, Contracting and the New Public Management.* Macmillan, Basingstoke.

Walt, G. (1994) *Health Policy: An Introduction to Process and Power.* Zed Books, London.

Walt, G. and Gilson, L. (1994) Reforming the health sector in developing countries: the central role of policy analysis. *Health Policy and Planning* 9: 353–70.

Walt, G., Pavignani, E., Gilson, L. and Buse, K. (1999) Managing external resources in the health sector: are there lessons for Swaps? *Health Policy and Planning* 14(3): 273–84.

Wanasinghe, S. (1994) Financing of health care in Sri Lanka: issues and options. Paper presented for the Symposium on the Design and Management of National Health Policies in Sri Lanka, Marga Institute, Colombo, 6–8 July.

Watkins, K. (forthcoming) Cost recovery and equity: the case of Zimbabwe. In Mwabu, G. Ugaz, C. and White, G. (eds) *New Patterns of Social Service Provision in Low Income Countries.* UNU/WIDER, Helsinki.

Weber, M. (1946) Bureaucracy. In Gerth, H.H. and Wright Mill, C. (eds). *From Max Weber: Essays in Sociology.* New York: Oxford University Press reprinted in *Public Policy: The Essential Readings*; eds. Stella Theodoulou and Matthew Cahn, Prentice Hall, 1995. p. 259–65.

Werna, E. (1995) *The Health Sector in Venezuela*. The Role of Government in Adjusting Economies Paper No. 5, University of Birmingham, Birmingham.

WHO (World Health Organisation) (1999) *The World Health Report 1999. Making a difference*. WHO, Geneva.

Wight, A.R. (1997) Participation, Ownership and Sustainable Development. In Grindle, M. (ed.) *Getting Good Government: Capacity Building in the Public Sectors of Developing Countries*. Harvard University Press, Cambridge, MA.

World Bank (1998) *Reducing Poverty in India: Options for More Effective Public Services*. World Bank, Washington DC.

World Bank (1997a) *The State in a Changing World: World Development Report 1997*. Oxford University Press, Oxford.

World Bank (1997b) *Financing Health Care: Issues and Options for China*. Washington, DC: World Bank China 2020 Series, Volume 4.

World Bank (1994) *India: Policy and Finance Strategies for Strengthening Primary Health Care Services*. The World Bank, Washington, DC.

World Bank (1993) *World Development Report 1993: Investing in Health*. Oxford University Press, New York.

World Bank (1987) *Financing Health Services in Developing Countries: An Agenda for Reform*. World Bank, Washington DC.

Yepes, F. and Sanchez, L.H. (in press) Reforming pluralist systems: the case of Colombia. In Mills, A. (ed.) *Reforming Health Sectors*. Kegan Paul, London.

Yesudian, C.A.K. (1994) Behaviour of the private sector in the health market in Bombay. *Health Policy and Planning* 9(1): 72–80.

Zwi, A. and Mills, A. (1995) Health policy in less developed countries: past trends and future directions. *Journal of International Development* 7(3): 299–328.

Index

Waiting times, 26
Weber, Max, 8, 65; *see also* bureaucracy
Western medicine
  consumer information on, 62
  as expression of state power, 43, 44;
    see also colonial state
World Bank, 51 58, 98, 201; *and see*
    under; structural adjustment
    programmes

Zimbabwe
  accounting system, 85
  bed occupancy rate, 33
  capacity constraints, 112–13
  church hospitals, 24, 44, 121, 134
  colonial legacy, 31
  contract policy, 121, 136, 135–7
  contracting out, 58, 121–2, 123–4, 218
  cost recovery, 109
  curative care, bias towards, 31, 45–6
  decentralisation, 55, 72; resistance to,
    84
  drug shortages, 34
  drug use, inefficient, 34
  Economic and Social Adjustment
    Programme, 51
  economic crisis, 98
  facility managers, 111

financial information system, 86
government capacity, 135–7
government health spending, 30;
  cuts in, 101
Health Professions Council, 165
Health Reform Agenda, 151
health sector reform, 58, 60;
  opposition to, 59
health status, 37
hospital autonomy, 72
informal care, 23
Medical Council, 164
Ministry of Health, role of, 59
not-for-profit insurance, 23, 62
preventive care, 46
primary care, 46
private sector, 146
regulatory legislation, 157
role of state, 43, 50
Salisbury Hospitals Act 1975, 72
skills shortages, 177
social development fund, 111
tertiary care, 45–6
traditional practitioners, 23
user fees, 101; effect on poor, 29, 102;
  exemptions, 111; pressure for,
  99; revenue generation, 100;
  revenue retention, 109